Daniel 1:8
"Daniel made up his mind.

D0558116

The Daniel Fast

A complete resource of guidelines,
menus, recipes, and spiritual journal

by **Annette Reeder**

Author of *Treasures of Healthy Living*

**with Rhonda Sutton
and Debbie Markwood**

ISBN: 978-0-9853969-4-7

We wish to thank the following for their time and devotion to making the recipes and taking the pictures for this cookbook:

Debra Brune	Joy Lloyd	Stacey Sutton
Tatiana Buchanan	Linda McKean	Tracy Wainwright
Patty Clark	Cheryl Morgan	Bonnie Witte
Ellen Lauer		

And Daniel made up his mind

Daniel 1:8

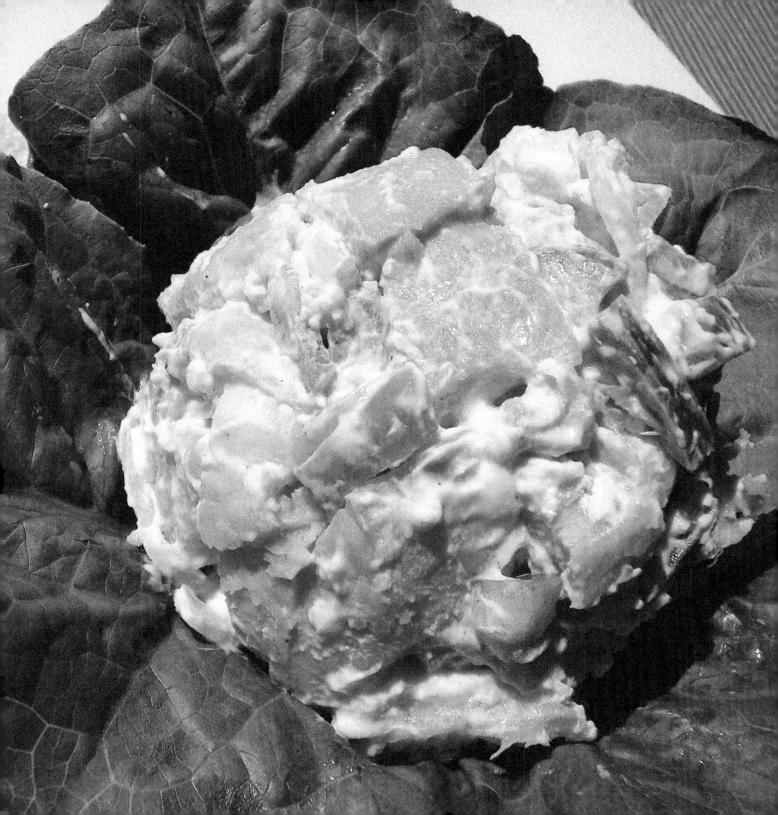

Contents

About the Authors

Annette Reeder, B.S. Nutrition, Professional member ASN and NANP, a Tour Guide to Biblical Health, is leading people all around the country on an adventure with the power of food to change lives one meal and prayer at a time. Her books, *Treasures of Healthy Living, Treasures of Health Nutrition Manual* and *Healthy Treasures Cookbook* are part of the tools to reach the ultimate health God desired. She is the founder of Designed Healthy Living a ministry aiming to bring the Biblical message of health to the church. Annette and her team are dedicated to changing lives one meal at a time through her writings, Flavor of Grace Conferences, Cooking Classes and Biblical Wellness Seminars.

> "I was greatly inspired by Annette's insightful, inspiring and challenging messages. She is knowledgeable on this much needed subject and is a lovey winsome lady, who out of great conviction presents valid reasons for following this healthy lifestyle."
>
> Joyce Rogers, author, speaker, and wife of the late Adrian Rogers

Rhonda Sutton, RN, BSN, MSN is passionate about teaching others to understand how the body works in order to promote health and well-being. She has taught in several colleges as a Nurse Educator for nearly 20 years. She has served as a missionary in France and also holds a Certificate in Biblical Counseling. Rhonda and her husband, Joel, are the parents of 3 grown children and make their home in Richmond, Virginia.

Debbie Markwood – Debbie was a tremendous help in outlining the recipes and contributing many from her own kitchen. It is a true delight to meet such wonderful people on this journey.

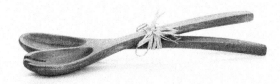

About Designed Healthy Living

Designed Healthy Living is on mission sharing the gift of health along with the treasures of wisdom and knowledge to understand what the Bible says about healthy living.

Changing lives ~ one meal at a time with these tools:

Treasures of Healthy Living Bible Study – Did you know you can find the answers to many health problems in the pages of Scripture? Think of God's Word as a treasure map that leads straight to the healthy life you've always dreamed of. It reveals how you can move from a sickly, lackluster life tone that is full of energy and hope. This practical Bible study will reveal the truth about the foods you eat and provide simple tools to begin improving your physical, emotional and spiritual heath. You won't believe how much your life can change when you grab hold of the treasures God has provided for you.

This book along with the full collection of the Treasures of Health Series can be found at www.DesignedHealthyLiving.com.

12 week DVD series; Leader Kit; Books; CD series; Homeschool Teacher Guide (These can all be found on the Designed Healthy Living website.)

Flavor of Grace Conferences – Spreading across the country, these conferences bring a fresh perspective on how Scripture and nutrition intimately coincide. Learn biblical principles to transform your health. Enjoy delicious cooking classes and be challenged to be a witness through your health.

Cooking Classes – Everyone loves food so why not bring a fun Flavor of Grace Cooking Class to your group, business or church? Learning biblical principles that can change your health will be an easy step once you taste the 'good' food God designed. All classes include: tasty samples, simple demonstrations, recipes to take home and lessons of God's beautiful design of our bodies.

Dreading Fasting Testimony

In the past, I tried several times to break unhealthy eating habits and start exercising, but I kept falling back into old routines. Last year after the Christmas holidays, I hit my highest weight ever, even counting being pregnant! In my quest for a healthier lifestyle, I decided to turn to the *Treasures of Healthy Living Bible Study.* I knew it was time for some "drastic measures" before my health paid a costly price. These problems were not going away or getting any easier to address with age and depleting estrogen on the horizon.

I enthusiastically embraced *The Treasures of Healthy Living Bible Study.* Everything was going well until I got to the chapter on fasting. Chapter 7 is safely hidden in the middle of the study! I was excited about my progress during the study up to this point, but the "fasting chapter" was such a high hurdle for me to face. I felt so overwhelmed at the thought of fasting for more than "just between meals" (no snacking between meals was a real accomplishment for me!). One question adequately described my feelings after reading this chapter, "Are you crazy?" I quickly went on to the next chapter not giving the "fasting chapter" serious consideration. I was not ready to do something so unusual.

Then it happened. The following week, it seemed that everywhere I went; I saw something about "fasting". The word was literally "popping out" at me on bookshelves. I prayed to the Lord and asked Him, "Are you trying to tell me something?" I knew that God wanted me to trust Him in all things. I sensed that He wanted me to fast and claim the victory by faith that I could fast successfully. He helped me to see that I could already claim by faith that He would give me the strength to fast. The Lord gave me the faith to view the Daniel Fast as a "done deal" even before I began the first day. He wanted me to walk with Him each step of the way in His power; I just had to cooperate with the Holy Spirit and depend on Him alone.

My mind, spirit, will, emotions and body started the amazing and purifying journey of fasting. My focus changed from food to feasting on the promises of God and His Word as I completed each day by the grace and strength of the Lord. The "Daniel Fast" transformed my fear and frustration to a new level of freedom and joy. I was able to pray with a clearer focus and ardent desire to please the Lord Jesus. I knew that the Holy Spirit was guiding me as I consecrated myself to Him in the way I treated my body, His temple. I began experiencing a new level of abundant living through Christ.

The only requirement for fasting is the commitment to trust the Lord in the most basic area: what we eat and drink. It is unfamiliar territory for many of us. Food is comfort. He is faithful and strong enough to supply all that we need to be obedient. I am so thankful that He would not let me skip over the wisdom and truth about fasting. I started seeing the lies that I had believed about food and what is really good for me. As I lost the weight, I also let go of fears and lies about food and exercise. I gained a new perspective about healthy food that I could fit into my schedule and the exercise that works best with my personality that I can maintain for the rest of my life.

I feel so much better now. I used to think that being "good" to myself revolved around eating comfort food. Now I know the truth about being really "good" to myself. The Lord knows what He is talking about. It just took me awhile to agree with Him about food and exercise. He wants us to be totally free in Christ. This includes food freedom. He used fasting to "wake me up" spiritually so that I would not miss out on His best for me. When I feel better physically, I want to do more for Him and my family. I have more energy and joy when I am following His plan for life instead of going my "own way". Fasting is not crazy. It is one avenue to freedom and joy for healthy living. I do not dread fasting, chapter 7 anymore.

Rhonda Sutton

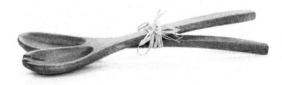

Steps to Fasting

Introduction

The purpose of a fast is freedom. Freedom to hear God in a new way as reliance on favorite foods is put aside. If the result is not greater freedom, then something is wrong. There will be times in your life when fasting is necessary to break the bonds of strongholds such as gossiping, alcohol, food addictions, lack of trust, sinful behaviors and so on. Turning your problems over to God and letting Him take control over these areas will bring this freedom and a great yoke will be lifted from your shoulders. Discipline always has its rewards. It will be difficult before it is easy.

For an in-depth study on fasting read Week 7 in the *Treasures of Healthy Living* Bible study (pages 186-203) and in the *Treasures of Health Nutrition Manual* (pages 259-265).

Before You Begin
Make up your mind:

To fast or not to fast is one question and the next question is why? There are several occasions of fasting in the book of Daniel, but one of my favorite stories is the one about Daniel and his friends Shadrach, Meshach and Abednego. Read Daniel 1.

Daniel and his friends were offered all the king's delicacies, yet they chose to eat a diet of vegetables. Daniel had proposed in his heart ahead of time that he would not defile himself. He avoided rich foods such as meats, pastries, cakes, cookies, alcohol and any other food that is tempting to the flesh. As you read about Daniel and his friends, the Scripture explains how they were much healthier than the other Hebrew teenagers. This form of fasting followed eating foods God declared good for you and not the foods altered or abused by man. Daniel's health was a testimony to God's provision. When we fast for physical well-being, God will touch our bodies and enrich our souls.

When considering a fast the first fast will not be easy. You will be more successful if you determine in your mind a head of time that you are going to do this. Then the other preparations will fall into place. If you make a mistake, start over.

Make a Commitment

God wants us to demonstrate our commitment to Him. Take the following steps to show Him your intent.

- Determine in your heart and mind that you are going to fast.

- Set a date – in advance and make a commitment. Commitment cards are at the back of this book; one for you and one for you to share with an accountability partner if you choose.

- Determine the spiritual reason for your fast. See page 193 in *Treasures of Healthy Living* for a list to review.

Make a Plan

Putting too many rules on a fast can be a distraction from the purpose. These guidelines listed here are just that – guidelines. It is up to each person to set their own parameters of how they want to implement a fast, especially the Daniel fast.

Daniel 1:12 *Please test your servants for ten days, and let us be given some vegetables to eat and water to drink.*

Daniel 10:2-3 *In those days I, Daniel, had been mourning for three entire weeks. I did not eat any tasty food, nor did meat or wine enter my mouth, nor did I use any ointment at all, until the entire three weeks were completed.*

These verses in Daniel give a brief synopsis of Daniel's food plan. The definition of vegetables is your discretion. It could literally be just vegetables alone or the word vegetables could include other foods such as fruits and grains.

In Daniel 10, it is up to you to decide again what he meant by tasty foods. Vegetables can be tasty. You decide what to eat and not eat. Don't let anyone put rules on you; it is between you and the LORD. It is clear Daniel did not eat any meat or drink wine. Listed here are some guidelines or suggestions.

Foods to include: All fruits, vegetables, whole grains, nuts and seeds, legumes, quality oils, pure water, herbal teas, soy products(high quality non-GMO), natural vinegars, seasonings, salt, herbs and spices.

Foods to avoid: All meat and animal products, dairy products, sweeteners, refined and processed food products, deep fried foods, solid fats, beverages other than pure water and herbal teas.

A meal plan and recipes are included in this book to make it easier during this special time with the Lord.

Make Time for Prayer and Meditation

Be careful, to take your mind off eating some people fill every waking moment with activity. Besides being in a continual mind of prayer throughout your day specific time needs to be set aside for prayer and meditation on God's Word. Without this scheduled time of prayer the fast becomes nothing more than abstinence from food. Read Isaiah 58. The spirit and body are so interrelated in God's creative design that fasting has both spiritual and physical benefits. By enabling us to surrender our lives to God in greater measure, we find fasting gives us more control over our tongues, our minds, our attitudes, our emotions, our bodies and all our fleshly desires. By setting this time for prayer while not eating it helps us submit our heart to God completely so that He can use us for His purpose.

In Isaiah 58 is a promise from God each time you fast. "Is not this the fast that I have chosen; to lose the bonds of wickedness." We all need deliverance from bondage and fasting accompanied by prayer will help break that bound of wickedness.

Just as you are setting a plan for the foods to eat, also set a time – or several times a day for specific prayer and reading God's Word.

Make Healthy Foods a Delight

Fasting does not need to be a struggle. Once you get past the first 12 hours it becomes easier to follow through with your commitment. Make God's food a delight instead of drudgery. Every good and perfect gift comes from God and this includes the best of foods imaginable. Learn new cooking techniques, new spices, marinades, new recipes. Each time you find a new food you love – give thanks. Make each day exciting as you venture out to new foods and undiscovered taste. This may be the most fabulous foodie experience you ever ventured.

Make Preparations

The day you start the Daniel Fast is not the day to write the menu and shopping list. Plan ahead. Once you set the date to begin and have written out your commitment, write out your menu. The menu in this book suggests ideas to help you through your first fast. A shopping list is also included.

Remove **all** tempting foods **now** before you begin. If you don't want to be wasteful then try freezing foods such as cheese, butter, milk, and meat. Eggs do not freeze but they do last a long time in the refrigerator. Throw away all cookies, ice cream, sweets, and other temptations. Set yourself up to succeed. Even though you are doing this for spiritual reasons don't even think you will not be tempted – you will. Satan will make sure of it. Remember we wrestle not against flesh and blood but against principalities. This means you are entering spiritual warfare and food will be used against you.

Make sure you have a good water purifier. There are better brands than Brita and Pur. Be a smart shopper.

Make Praises

As your feet hit the floor each morning give a shout of rejoicing for the great insight God will give you today. Continue to praise Him all the day long and especially at the end of this short journey.

This is the day that the Lord has made, let us rejoice and be glad in it. Psalm 118:24

Meal Ideas

The following recipes can be found in the *Healthy Treasures Cookbook* on the page numbers indicated. If no page number is listed, the recipe is included in this book in alphabetical order. These recipes are hyperlinked (in the download version) so you can find them easily. Many recipes in the *Healthy Treasures Cookbook* or your own favorite cookbook can be easily adapted into the Daniel Fast by omitting ingredients to be avoided and substituted with allowed ingredients. An example of soups; substitute chicken broth with vegetable broth.

These recipes were compiled with the assistance of Debbie Markwood at Colonial Heights Baptist Church. Debbie is a beautiful example of living and enjoying the foods God designed.

Breakfast

- Breakfast Burritos

- Chewy Breakfast Bars

- Cream of Wheat: page 21 (use rice or almond milk and heat with dates for a sweetener)

- Fruit

- Muesli Mix: page 26

- Muesli-Nut Fruit Salad: page 25 (*omit yogurt and use fruit juice, water or almond milk to make cold or hot cereal*)

- Nuts

- Oats: Overnight Oatmeal, Cherry Berry Muesli

- Pancakes

- Surprise Berry Juice

Lunch/Side Dishes/Salads

- Any fruit
- Any vegetables
- Black Bean Salad: page 143 (*use seasoned oil & vinegar instead of Italian dressing*)
- Black Bean Soup: page 125 (use vegetable broth and omit sour cream)
- Blackberry Mixed Salad: page 144
- Chickpea Salad: page 75
- Classic Carrot Soup: page 130
- Green Salads
- Grilled Summer Squash & Tomatoes: page 78
- Italian Chickpeas : page 76
- Lentil Salad: page 154
- Lentil Soup
- Oven Baked Butternut Squash: page 79
- Quinoa Pilaf: page 163
- Roasted Sweet Potatoes: page 80
- Stir Fry Zucchini: page 82
- Sweet Potato Salad
- Tabouli (Wheat Garden Salad): page 172
- Tuscan White Bean Salad
- Vegetable Soup
- Vegetarian Stew
- Zesty Rice & Bean Salad

Dinner/Soup

- Bean and Rice Casserole
- Bean Burgers & Salsa
- Bean Curry and Rice
- Black Bean Soup: page 125 (omit yogurt and use vegetable instead of chicken broth)
- Black Beans and Rice
- Cabbage Rolls
- Italian Tomato Bean Soup
- Italian Vegetables Soup: page 132
- Lentil-Barley Stew: page 133
- Marinated Vegetable Salad
- Nice & Nutty Veggie Burgers
- Popeye Burgers
- Quinoa Pilaf
- Soup recipes can be adapted to the fast by using water or vegetable base instead of meat stock/broth
- Spanish Paella
- Spelt Chapatti: page 112
- Stir Fry Vegetables with Brown Rice
- Sweet Potato Pie
- Taco Soup: page 136
- Three Bean Indian Dal
- Turkish Salad

- Tuscan Villa Bean Soup

- Vegetable Pizza

- Vegetable Soup: your favorite recipe made with a vegetable base instead of meat stock/broth

- Vegetarian Chili

- Vegetarian Stew

- Veggie Medley/ Pasta

- Veggie Wraps

Snacks

- Crispy Beans

- Corn Chips

- Fruit – fresh or dried

- Nuts

- Popcorn – no butter

- Trail mix of nuts, dry fruit, seeds, coconut

- Veggies

Breads

- Chapattis or Indian Flat Bread

- Homemade Crackers

- Israelite Unleavened Bread

Daniel Fast 21-Day Menu

Day	Pg.	Breakfast	Pg.	Lunch	Pg.	Dinner	Pg.	Snack
1	CB 26	Muesli w/ Almond milk, sliced fruit		Steamed Vegetables with brown rice; apple	DF	Vegetarian Chili, Green Salad w/vinaigrette, orange slices	CB 3	Bean Hummus with raw cauliflower, carrots, peppers
2	CB 190-199	Fruit Smoothie Ezekiel Bread toast	DF	Vegetarian Chili; carrot & celery sticks	DF	Nutty Veggie Burgers w/bean Mango Salsa; Oven-Roasted Broccoli; Apple Slices	CB 5	Black Bean Dip with Carrot Sticks
3	CB 24	Overnight Oatmeal; flavored with raisins, dates, apples, cinnamon, vanilla	CB 154	Lentil Salad; orange slices	CB 136	Taco Soup (subst. Bulgur wheat for meat); green salad with vinaigrette; Corn Chips	CB 229	Dried Fruit Balls
4	CB 24	Fruitful Rice Pudding (omit honey)	CB 136	Taco Soup served over brown rice; serving of fresh fruit	DF CB 43	Three-Bean Indian Dal; green salad w/ oil & vinegar; Israelite Unleavened Bread w/Olive Oil Dipping Sauce		Frozen Grapes
5	CB 31	Chewy Breakfast Bars; apple	DF	Tuscan White Bean Salad; fresh fruit	CB 163 112	Quinoa Pilaf, Spelt Chapatti with herb dipping oil	CB 3	Hummus with vegetable plate

Day	Pg.	Breakfast	Pg.	Lunch	Pg.	Dinner	Pg.	Snack
6		Toast spread with 1 T. peanut or almond butter; banana	CB 163	Quinoa Pilaf, celery and carrot sticks	DF	Daniel Fast Cabbage Rolls; Frozen Grapes		Fruit plate; almonds
7		Oatmeal Make your own variety	CB 176	Zesty Rice & Bean Salad (omit feta cheese); Oven Roasted Broccoli	CB 132 DF	Italian Vegetable Soup; Turkish Salad; crackers	DF	Krunchy Kale Krisps
8	DF	Yummy Brown Rice w/Apple	CB 132	Vegetable Soup, green salad w/ vinaigrette	CB 50, 104 153	Vegetable Pizza, Fall Harvest Salad	DF	White Bean Dip w/ carrots & celery
9		Fruit Smoothies	CB 130	Classic Carrot Soup (omit honey); Sweet Brown Rice with Spicy Sauce	DF	Vegetable Fried Rice; fruit plate		Frozen Grapes
10	CB 22-23	Pancakes with fruit sauce		Steamed Vegetables with Quinoa; apple or fruit of choice	CB	Veggie wraps, green salad with vinaigrette, orange slices	CB 208	Healthy Banana Cookies
11		Surprise Delight Juice	DF	Vegetable Fried Rice Wraps	DF	Tuscan Villa Bean Soup; mixed green salad	CB 2	Hummus w/ veggies

Day	Pg.	Breakfast	Pg.	Lunch	Pg.	Dinner	Pg.	Snack
12	CB 31	Chewy Breakfast Bars; apple slices	DF	Tuscan Vila Bean Soup; carrot sticks	DF	Veggie Medley Tomato Sauce over whole wheat pasta; Oven Roasted Broccoli and Cauliflower		Vegetable plate with almonds
13	CB 24	Fruitful Rice Pudding	DF	Veggie Medley Pizza	DF	Moroccan Vegetarian Stew; green salad		Fruit Plate; walnuts
14	DF	Dried Fruit Muesli w/ almond milk; sliced banana	CB 128 CB 172	Butternut Squash Soup Tabouli – Stuffed in Tomatoes	CB 54	Marinated Vegetable salad; fresh fruit; bread	DF	White Bean Dip w/ carrots & celery
15	CB 24	Overnight Oatmeal	CB 154	Marinated vegetable salad; mixed green salad	DF CB 158	Sweet Potato Pie; green salad; Mideast Pilaf		Frozen Grapes
16	CB 22-23	Pancakes, fruit topping	CB 136	Lentil Soup; celery w/ peanut butter	DF	Better Bean Burgers w/ Bean Mango Salsa; Kale Slaw; fruit slices	CB 229	Dried Fruit Balls
17	CB 193	Very Berry Drink; Toast	CB 75 112 43	Chickpea Salad, Spelt Chapatti w/ Olive Oil dipping oil	DF	Spanish Paella; tossed green salad	DF	Crispy Beans ; fruit slices

Day	Pg.	Breakfast	Pg.	Lunch	Pg.	Dinner	Pg.	Snack
18	CB 21	Cream of Wheat/ Almond Milk, sweeten w/ applesauce	DF	Tex Mex Chili: green salad; fresh fruit	DF	Italian Tomato Bean Soup; salad; organic corn chips	CB 3	Hummus with veggies
19		Cherry Berry Muesli	CB 125	Black Bean Soup; Tomato Walnut Salad	CB 132	Turkish Salad; Vegetable Soup	CB 208	Healthy Banana Cookies
20	190-199	Fruit Smoothie	DF	Savory Stuffed Peppers; veggie slices	DF	Daniel Fast Cabbage Rolls; fruit slices		Fruit plate; almonds
21	DF	Breakfast Burrito	DF	Sweet Potato Salad; fruit slices	DF	Popeye Burgers; green salad, fruit platter	DF	Krunchy Kale Krisps

Grocery Shopping List

Beverages

Milk – Rice, Almond, Organic Soy

Juice – fresh squeezed or juiced is the best choice; second best is organic with no sugar or sweetener added; last choice but not preferred are regular juice; orange, pineapple, lime, lemon

Butter Spreads

Almond Butter

Apple Butter – little or no sugar

Whole Grains

Brown rice

Bulgur wheat

Millet

Oats – old fashioned, quick, steel cut

Quinoa

Shredded coconut

Wheat

Nuts/ Seeds – raw

Almonds, walnuts, pecans, pine nuts

Sesame seeds, Flax Seeds, sunflower seeds

Beans – dried or canned

Black

Cannelloni

Garbanzo

Kidney

Lentils – any variety

Pinto beans

Baking Aisle

Almond extract

Baking powder, soda

Chili powder

Cinnamon

Coriander

Cumin

Dried minced onions, unless using fresh

Garlic powder, unless using fresh

Nutmeg

Olive oil

Oregano

Sesame Oil

Stevia

Vanilla extract

Whole wheat flour – fresh milled is best

Dressings
Apple Cider Vinegar (Braggs is best)

Braggs Liquid Aminos (yellow label, possibly in organic aisle)

Dijon Mustard

Ranch dressing mix, recipe to make your own in CB

Red wine vinegar

Taco seasoning, recipe to make your own in DF

Vinaigrette dressing, recipe to make your own in CB & DF

Wine vinegar

Dried Fruit
Apricots

Blueberries

Cranberries

Dates

Pitted prunes

Raisins

Canned Vegetables/Fruit – no sweetener added
Crushed pineapple

Diced tomatoes

Mexican tomatoes

Olives

Tomato sauce

Soup
Vegetable broth

Fresh Vegetables – be creative
Broccoli

Carrots

Cauliflower

Celery

Cucumbers

Eggplant

Garlic cloves

Ginger root – small amount

Green beans

Green cabbage

Green onions

Kale

Mushrooms

Onions

Peppers

Red onion

Red or purple potatoes

Salad greens

Spinach

Sweet potatoes

Tomatoes

Zucchini

Fresh Fruit – all varieties

Apples

Banana

Cantaloupe

Mango

Oranges

Peaches

Strawberries

Fresh Herbs (dried – optional)

Basil

Cilantro

Mint

Oregano

Parsley

Sage

Extras

Applesauce

Bread Crumbs

Cornmeal

Elbow macaroni

Hummus – or make your own

Protein Powder – must be organic, non-GMO

Tahini

Whole wheat tortillas

Freezer Section

Frozen fruit – all varieties

Frozen organic corn

Peas

Spinach

RECIPES

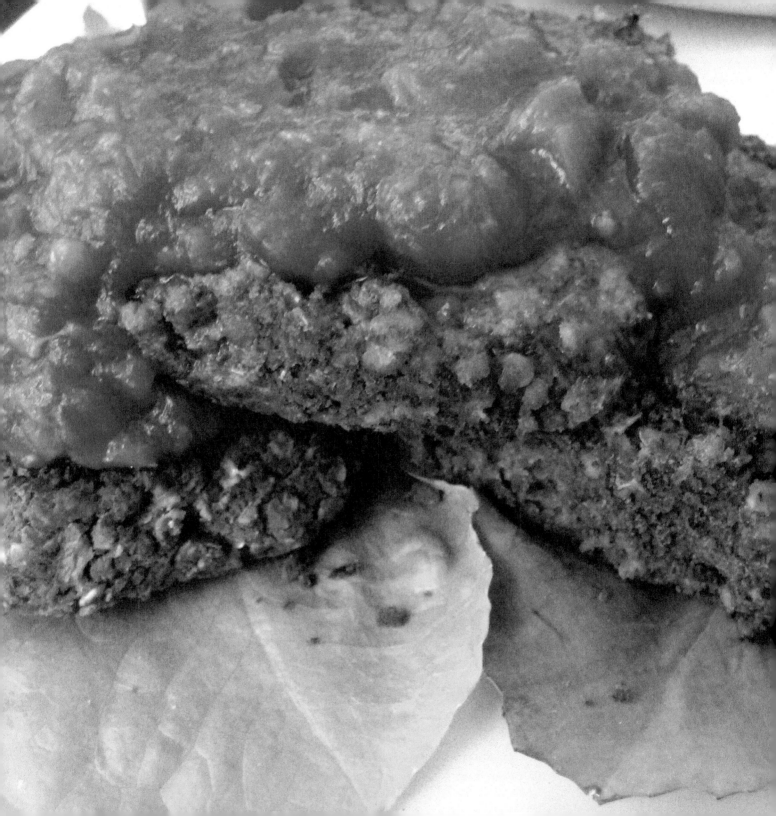

Better Bean Burgers

Ingredients:

- 3 cups cooked kidney or black beans
- 1 to 2 medium garlic cloves, finely chopped
- 3 tablespoons tomato paste
- 1 tablespoon red wine or balsamic vinegar
- 1 teaspoon Dijon mustard
- 3/4 cup green onions, sliced – green tops and white onion
- 1/4 cup fresh parsley, chopped
- 2 tablespoons fresh oregano, chopped (substitute 1 1/2 – 2 tsp. dried oregano)
- 1/2 teaspoon sea salt
  Black pepper to taste
- 1 1/4 cups rolled oats
- 1/2 cup organic corn
- 1/3 cup olives, chopped, optional
- 1/4 cup diced red bell pepper (optional)

Servings: 6-7 patties

In a food processor or blender, combine the beans, garlic, tomato paste, vinegar, and mustard. Pulse until pureed. Add the green onions, parsley, oregano, salt, and pepper to taste, and process to break up and blend. Add the oats and pulse to begin to incorporate. Transfer the mixture to a large bowl and stir in the olives, corn and red pepper.

Refrigerate the mixture for 30 to 45 minutes, then shape into patties with your hands.

*Skillet Option: Lightly coat skillet with oil and cook on medium/ medium-high heat.

Cook the patties for 6 to 8 minutes per side, or until golden brown.

*Oven Option: Bake the patties for about 15-20 minutes at 400 ° on an oiled pan, flipping once through cooking.

Delicious if topped with salsa or guacamole

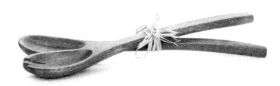

Black Bean and Mango Salsa

Ingredients:

- 1   cup black beans – cooked
- 2   mangos – peeled, seeded and finely diced
- ½   med. red pepper – cored, seeded, diced
- ½   med, green pepper – cored, seeded, diced
- ¾   cup pineapple juice
- ½   cup lime juice
- ½   cup fresh cilantro – chopped
- 2   tablespoons ground cumin
- 1   small jalapeno Chile pepper – seeded, minced
-     Salt and pepper – to taste

Servings: 5-8

Combine all ingredients in medium bowl. Adjust seasoning as desired.

Cover and refrigerate at least 1 hour or up to 4 days.

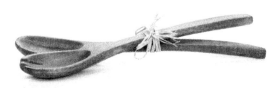

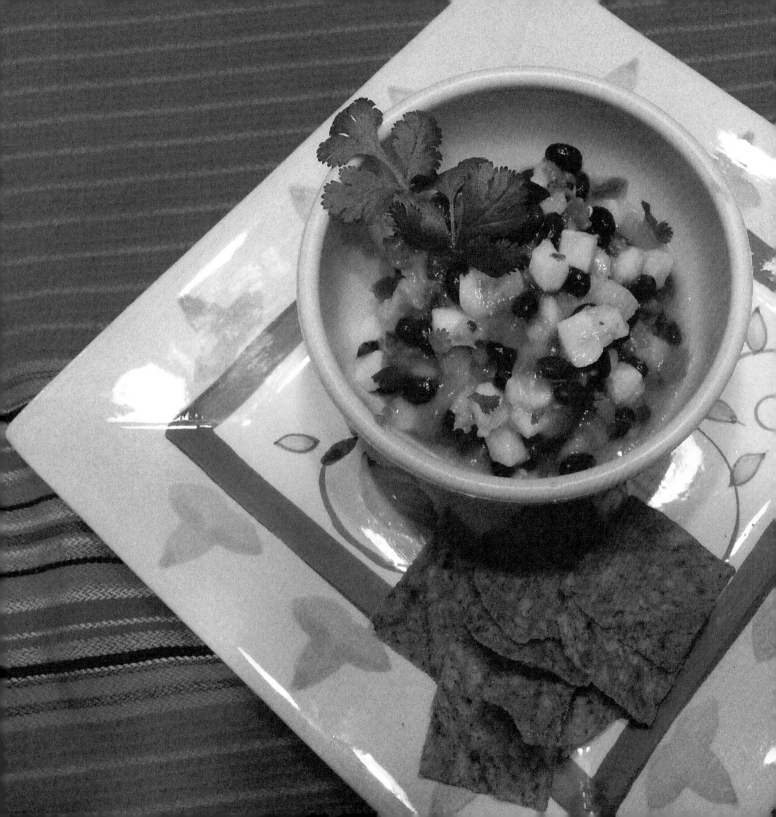

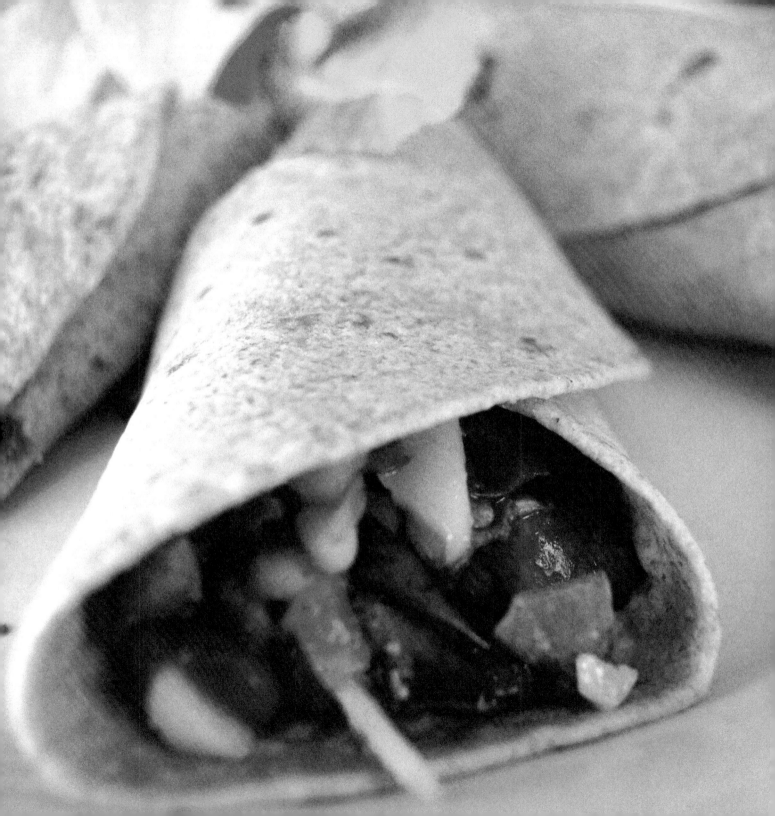

Breakfast Burrito

Ingredients:

½ cup red bell pepper, seeded and finely chopped

3 green onions, diced

2 cloves garlic, minced or pressed

⅓ cup water

2 cups red or black beans

1½ teaspoon Braggs Liquid Aminos

1 medium tomato, chopped

Herb seasoning mix – your favorite

5 ounces fresh spinach – coarsely chopped

6 tablespoons freshly ground flaxseeds

¼ cup soy cheese

Ezekiel Sprouted Grain Tortillas – or your favorite tortilla

Servings: 6

Recipe from: *The Antioxidant Diet*; Robin Jeep and Dr. Couey

In a large skillet, sauté peppers, onion and garlic in 1/3 cup water for 5 minutes. Add the beans and Bragg, cooking for another 5 minutes. Remove from heat and mix in tomatoes, seasoning or salt, spinach, flaxseed and soy cheese. Lightly toast the tortillas and stuff with bean filling.

This makes a great hot or cold sandwich filling for wraps or stuffed in a whole-wheat pita.

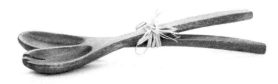

Cherry Berry Muesli

Ingredients:

½ cup oats – steel cut or old fashioned

½ cup pomegranate juice

1 banana, sliced

1 cup blueberries (fresh or frozen and thawed)

1 granny Smith apple – chopped

2 tablespoons ground flaxseed

¼ cup almond milk

3 tablespoons nonfat soy yogurt

2 tablespoons chopped raw nuts or
2 tablespoons sunflower seed butter

Servings: 2

Soak oats overnight in pomegranate juice.

Add other ingredients, mix and serve.

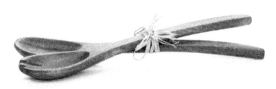

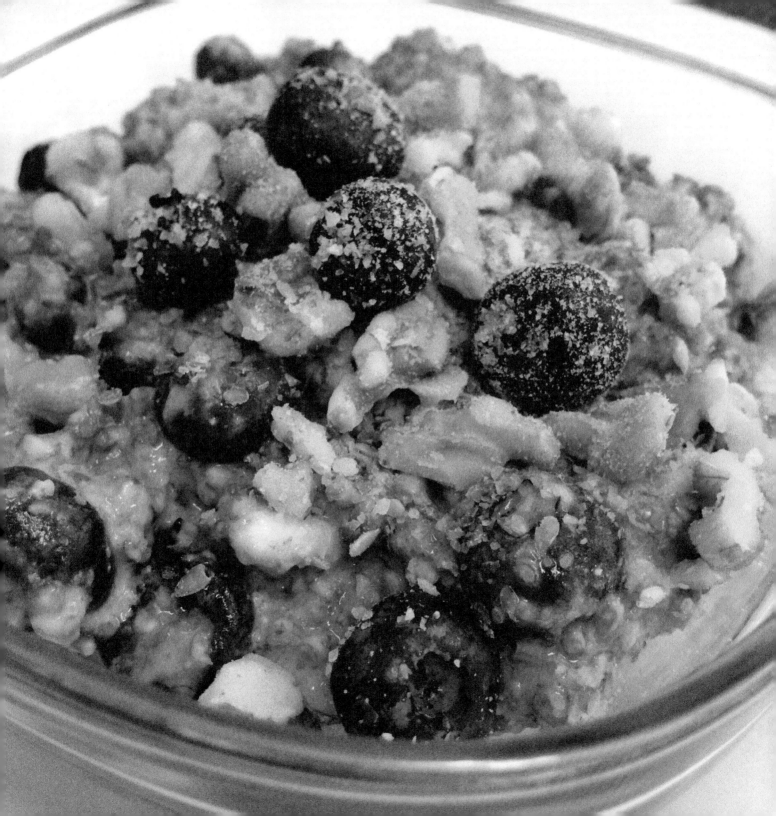

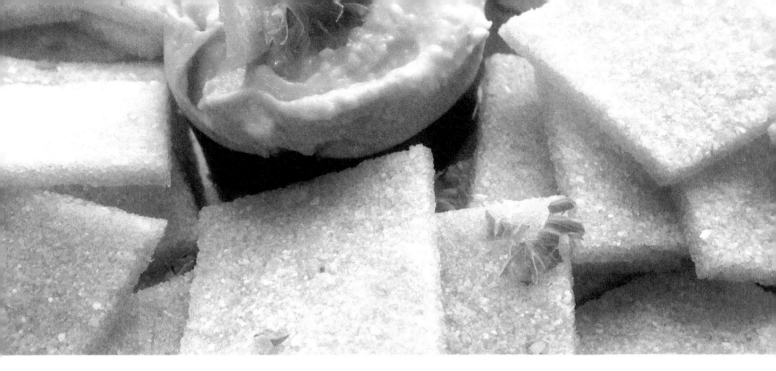

Corn Chips

Ingredients:

1   cup ground organic corn meal

1   tablespoon extra-virgin olive oil

$^1/_2$ teaspoon salt

$^3/_4$ cup boiling water

Servings: 8

Mix ingredients together. If dough is too dry add a little more water. Grease flat baking pan or stone. Dough will stick to rolling pin, so use a little bit of corn flour on pin as well as dough.

Roll very thin! Cut into squares and salt dough.

Bake 400 ° 8 minutes, remove pan & flip chips, bake 2 more minutes.

Remove from pan. Yields 1 lb. Store in airtight container or zip lock bag.

Note: Serve with your favorite hummis.

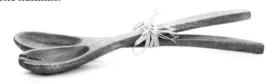

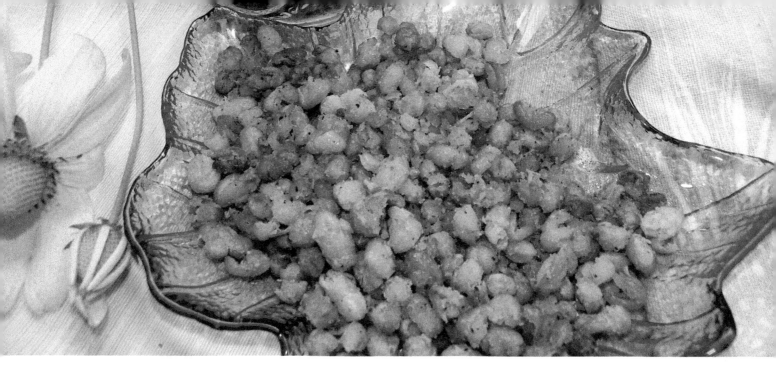

Crispy Beans

Ingredients:

1   can or 2 cups White Kidney Beans (or any bean of your choice)
     Olive oil
     Salt
     Pepper
     Rosemary

Rinse the beans. Spread on baking sheet and pat dry with paper towel. Drizzle with olive oil and stir until all are lightly coated. Season with salt, pepper and rosemary. Other spices would be good – be creative. Mix until well coated and seasoning are well distributed.

Bake in the oven at 450° for 25-30 minutes, until browned and crispy.

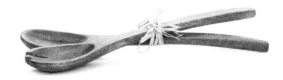

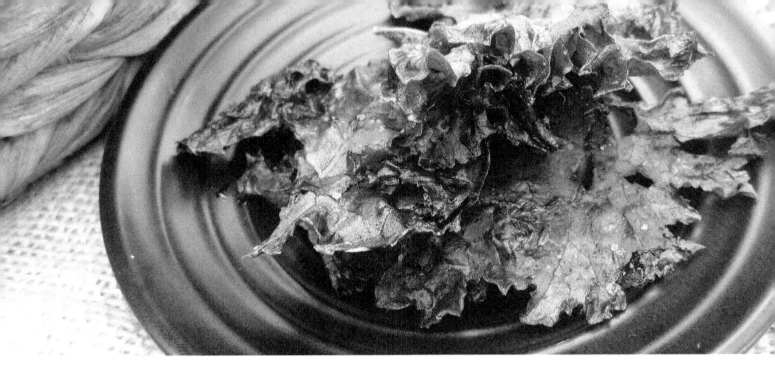

Krunchy Kale Krisps

Ingredients:

6   cups kale – rinsed, stems removed

1   tablespoon apple cider vinegar

2   tablespoons olive oil

½   teaspoon salt

Servings: 8

Preheat oven to 350 °. Cut the kale leaves in 2-3 inch pieces.

Combine the vinegar, oil, and salt in a large bowl; add the kale and toss by hand to make sure all leave are covered.

Place leaves in single layer on baking sheet and bake until they are crispy, about 20 minutes.

Check after 20 minutes, if they are not crispy, put back in oven and check after every 5 minutes. Remove when all leaves are crisp.

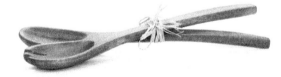

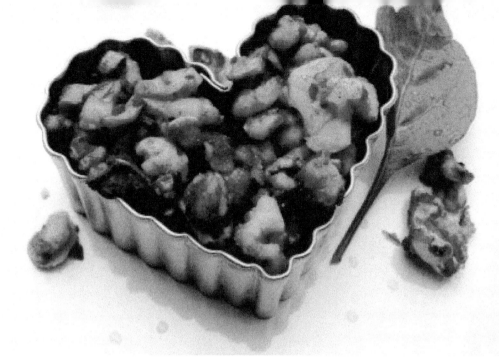

Cumin Roasted Walnuts

Ingredients:

2	cups walnuts – coarsely chopped
6	cloves garlic – minced or pressed
2	tablespoons olive oil
2	tablespoons ground cumin
1	tablespoon cumin seed
1	teaspoon sea salt
2	tablespoons honey

Serving Size: 16

Toast walnuts at 325 ° for 8-10 minutes.

Heat oil in medium skillet. Sauté garlic until golden. Stir in ground cumin, cumin seed, salt and honey.

Add toasted walnuts to skillet. Stir well to coat.

Spread evenly on baking sheet and bake at 375 ° for 20 minutes or until golden. Cool thoroughly.

Yield: 2 cups

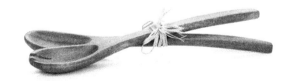

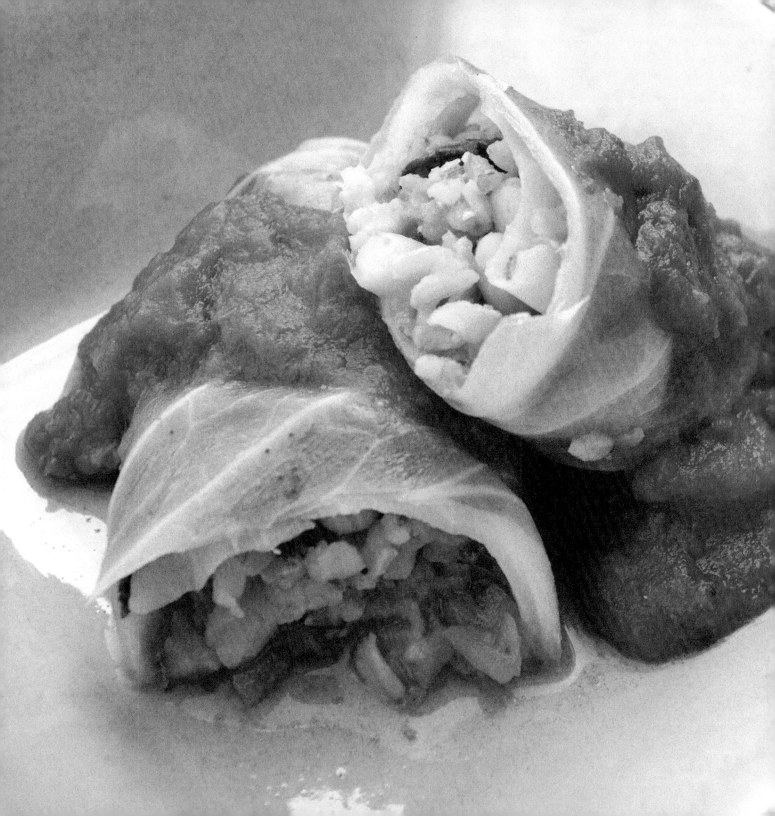

Daniel Fast Cabbage Rolls

Ingredients:

12	large cabbage leaves – regular or Napa
2	tablespoons olive oil
½	pound mushrooms – sliced
1	cup chopped onion
1	cup cooked brown rice
2	cups white beans
1	cup shredded carrot
2	tablespoons chopped parsley
1	teaspoon crushed oregano
½	teaspoon salt
¼	teaspoon pepper
8	ounces tomato sauce
1	teaspoon Italian herbs

Serving Size: 6

Preheat oven to 350 °.

Bring a large pot of water to boil; cook cabbage leaves, a few at a time for about 2 minutes or until softened. Drain and cool.

Heat oil over medium heat in a large skillet; sauté mushrooms and onion until tender.

Add rice, beans, carrot, parsley, oregano, salt and pepper; stir gently until well blended.

Prepare a shallow 2-quart baking dish by brushing with vegetable oil.

Spoon mixture onto individual cabbage leaves; roll up and place seam-side down on baking dish.

Cover with foil and bake at 350 ° for 30 minutes.

Heat tomato sauce and Italian herbs in a small saucepan, stirring often to prevent sticking.

Serve cabbage rolls with heated sauce.

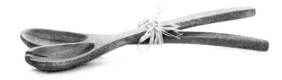

Hot and Spicy Hummus

Ingredients:

3	cups cooked garbanzo beans
1	cup tahini
¼	cup lemon juice
3	cloves garlic – crushed
½	teaspoon white pepper
1	teaspoon sea salt
1	teaspoon ground cumin
½	teaspoon red pepper flakes
½	teaspoon cayenne pepper
½	teaspoon black pepper
¼	cup jalapeno Chile peppers – finely diced

Puree garbanzo beans, tahini, and lemon juice until smooth, adding water as need to make a creamy mixture. Pour into a medium bowl.

Add remaining ingredients and stir well.

Chill to allow flavors to blend.

Yield: 4 cups

Serving Ideas: Serve as a dip with raw veggies or add to a tossed salad as a dressing.

This hummus is great in a whole grain wrap with lettuce, tomato and bean sprouts.

Comments: The red pepper flakes, cayenne and jalapenos can be omitted or cut in half if you prefer less spicy.

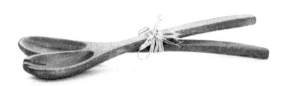

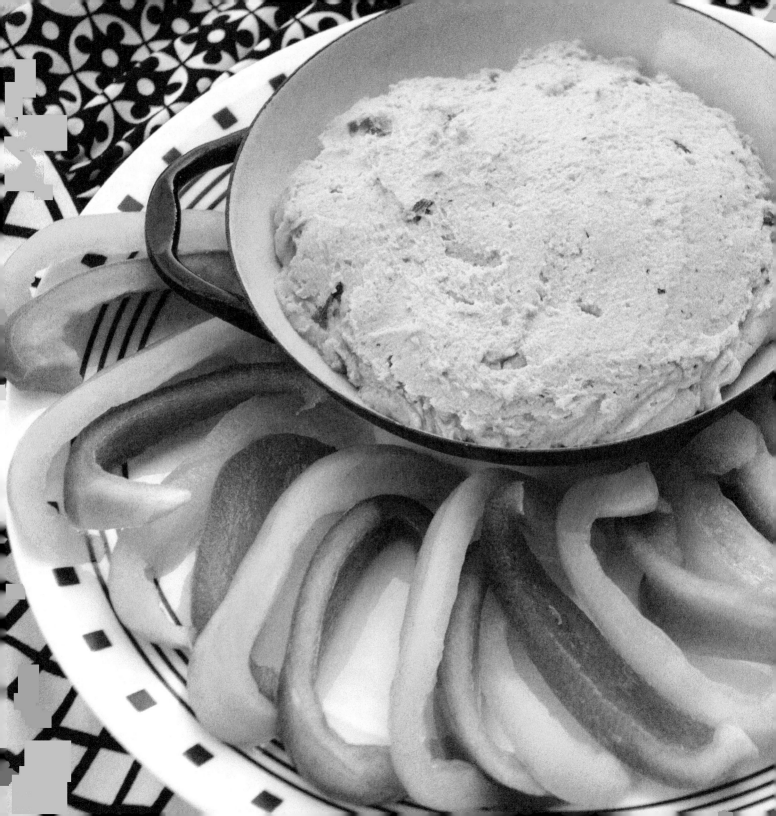

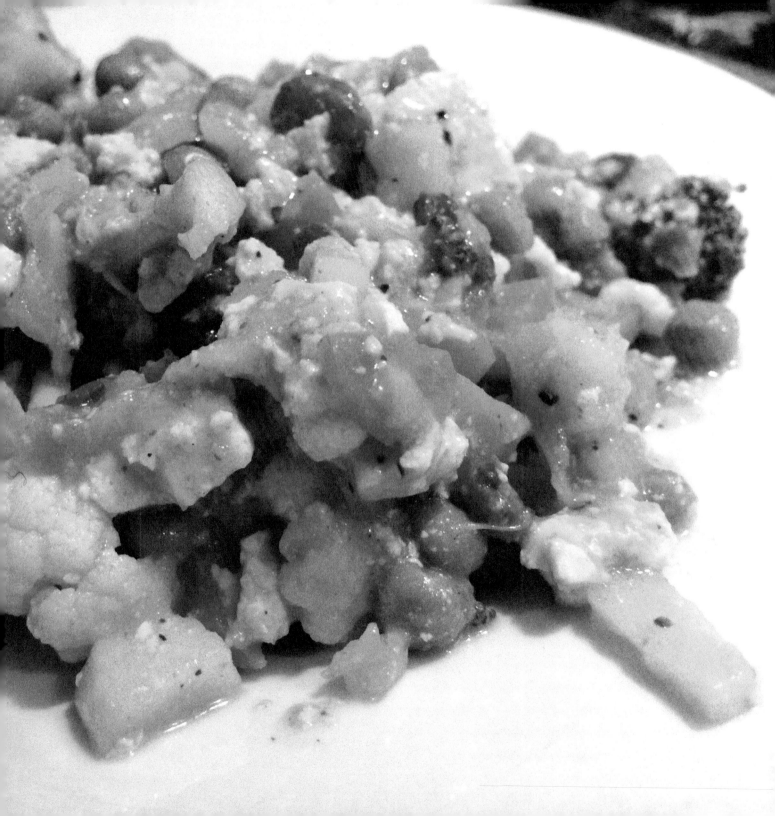

Indian Vegetable Curry

Ingredients:

1	tablespoon light sesame oil
1	cup onion – diced
2	cloves garlic – minced
1	teaspoon ground cumin
1	teaspoon sea salt
1	teaspoon black pepper
1	tablespoon curry powder
2	tablespoons fresh ginger – grated
2	tablespoons whole wheat flour
2	cups water
1	cup broccoli florets
1	cup cauliflower flowerets
½	cup chopped carrots
½	cup fresh green peas – frozen, organic will work
½	cup apple -- diced
½	cup raisins
1	cup firm tofu – cubed (see notes) *Must be organic, non GMO

Serving Size: 6

Heat oil in a large skillet and sauté onion and garlic until golden. Be careful not to burn the garlic. Add cumin, salt pepper, curry and ginger.

Stir in flour and cook 2-3 minutes. Slowly add water and mix until creamy and smooth.

Add broccoli, cauliflower, carrots, peas, apple, raisins and tofu, and cook until mixture is thick and bubbly and vegetables are tender.

Comments: If you like you may use 1 cup cooked garbanzo beans instead of the tofu.

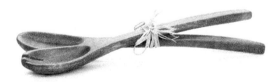

Kale Slaw

Ingredients:

1   bunch Fresh kale
1   large carrot – grated
½   orange – juiced
½   lemon – juiced
½   red onion – sliced
    Salt and pepper – to taste
1   tablespoon olive oil
1   tablespoon mayonnaise (Soy, or other
    vegan type mayo)
    *(Or 1 T. Olive oil plus 1 tsp. lemon juice
    may be substituted)*

Serving Size: 4

Place the kale into a salad bowl. Toss with the carrot, orange juice, lemon juice, and salt, and using your hands, rub the juice into the kale. Let the kale sit a few minutes while you prepare the onion.

Prepare a large bowl of ice water and a saucepan with boiling water. Place the thinly sliced onion into the boiling water for 15 to 30 seconds, and then shock them in the cold water, stopping the cooking immediately.

Drain the water and blot the onions with a paper towel. Add the onion, olive oil, salt and pepper and toss well. Add the mayonnaise and mix the slaw well.

Refrigerate until ready to serve.

Can be made several hours in advance.

Comments: Garnish with sunflower seeds, pine nuts, or nuts of your choosing.

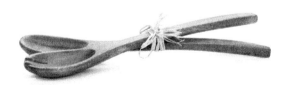

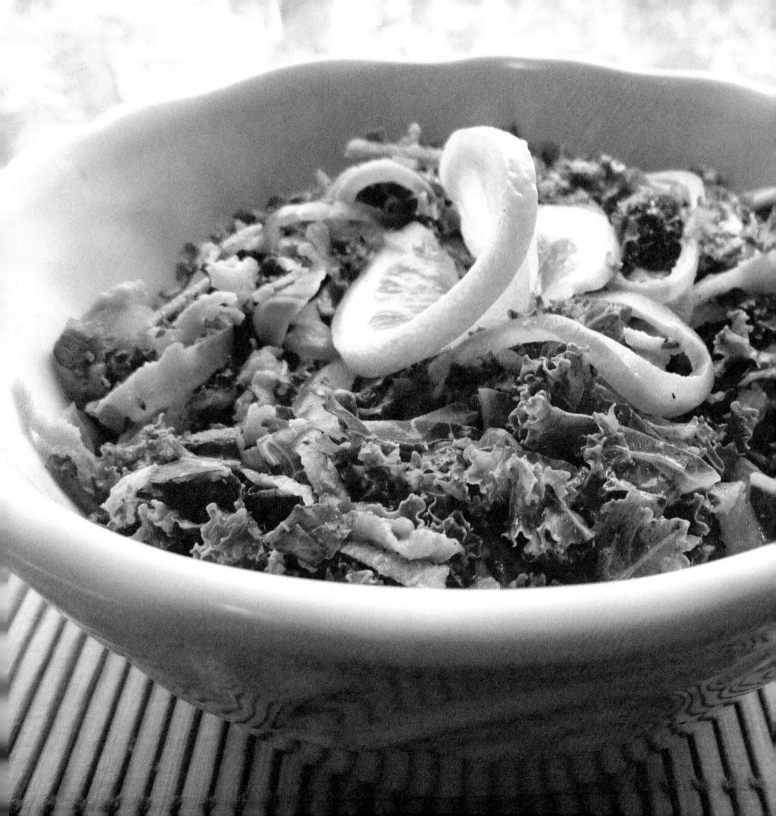

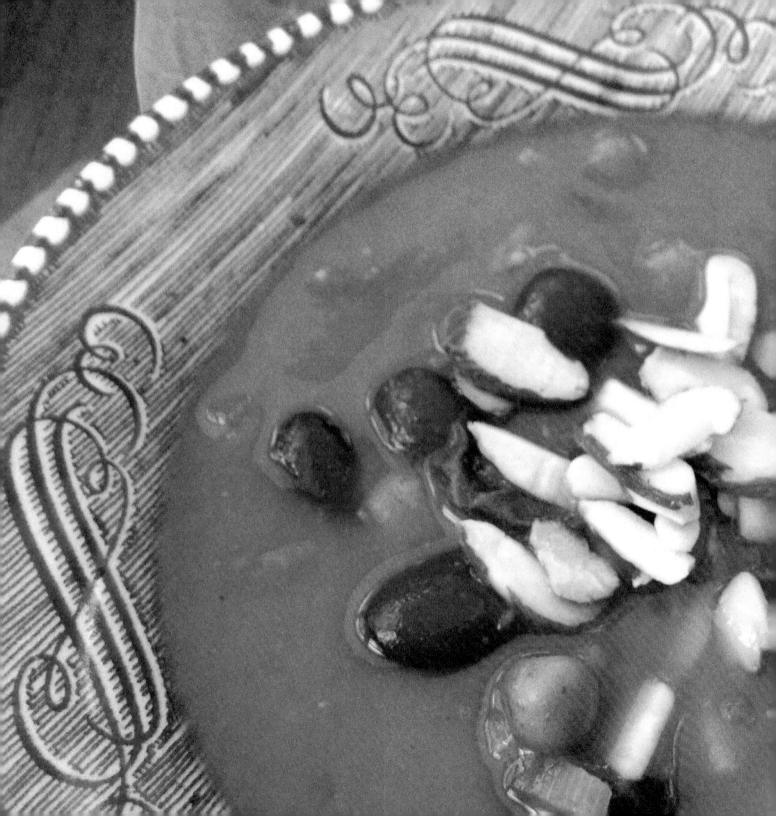

Fast Italian Tomato-Bean Soup

Ingredients:

4	cups organic tomato soup or Roasted Red Pepper soup
4	cups frozen spinach
4	cups chopped broccoli
1	cup fresh onion – chopped
2	cups frozen peas or green beans
2	cups diced tomatoes
3	cups carrot juice
2	garlic – minced
2	teaspoons dried Italian seasoning
2-3	cups red beans – cooked
4	tablespoons pine nuts or walnuts

Servings: 10

Recipe from *The Antioxidant Diet;* Robin Jeep and Dr. Couey

In a large pot, combine all ingredients except beans and nuts and simmer for 40 minutes. Add beans and simmer 10 additional minutes. Serve topped with nuts.

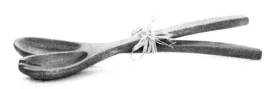

Mexican Bean Salad

Ingredients:

1	tablespoon olive oil
1/4	cup jalapeno Chile peppers – finely diced
2	cloves garlic – crushed
1/2	cup yellow onion – finely chopped
1	teaspoon sea salt
1	teaspoon black pepper
1/2	cup diced green bell pepper
1	cup diced tomatoes
1/2	teaspoon cayenne
1	teaspoon chili powder
1/4	cup chopped cilantro
1	cup cooked black beans
1	cup cooked kidney beans
1	cup cooked pinto beans
1/4	cup red wine vinegar – or lemon juice

Serving Size: 4

In a medium skillet, heat oil and sauté hot green pepper, garlic, onion, salt and black pepper until onion is translucent.

Stir in diced green pepper, tomatoes, cayenne, chili powder, and cilantro, and heat just until cilantro begins to wilt.

Turn tomato and pepper mixture into a medium mixing bowl. Add all of the beans and the vinegar (or lemon juice). Mix well and chill thoroughly before serving.

Serve on a bed of field greens or green leafy lettuce.

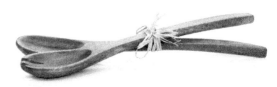

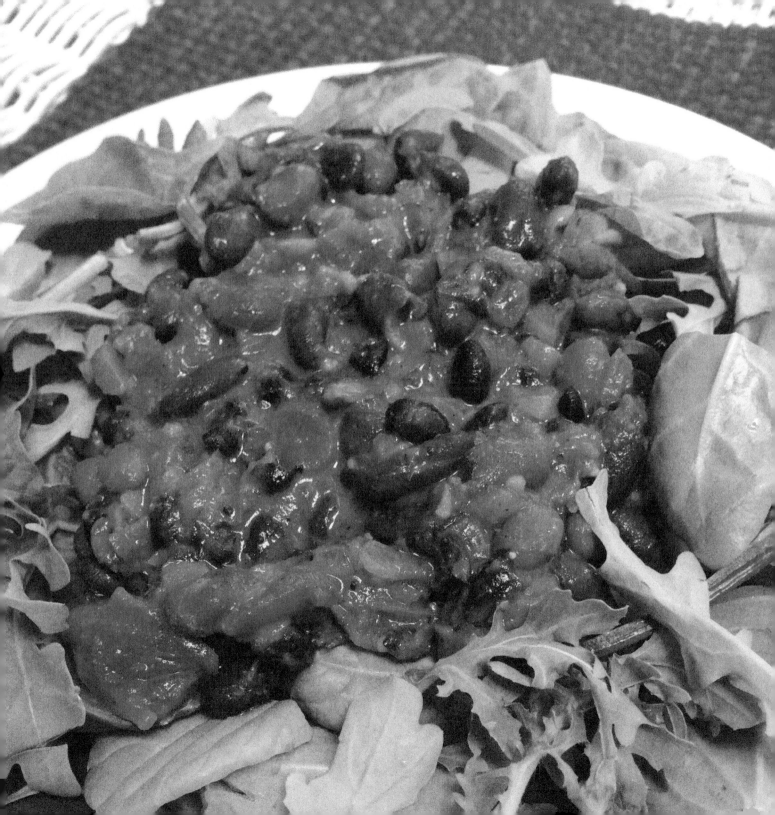

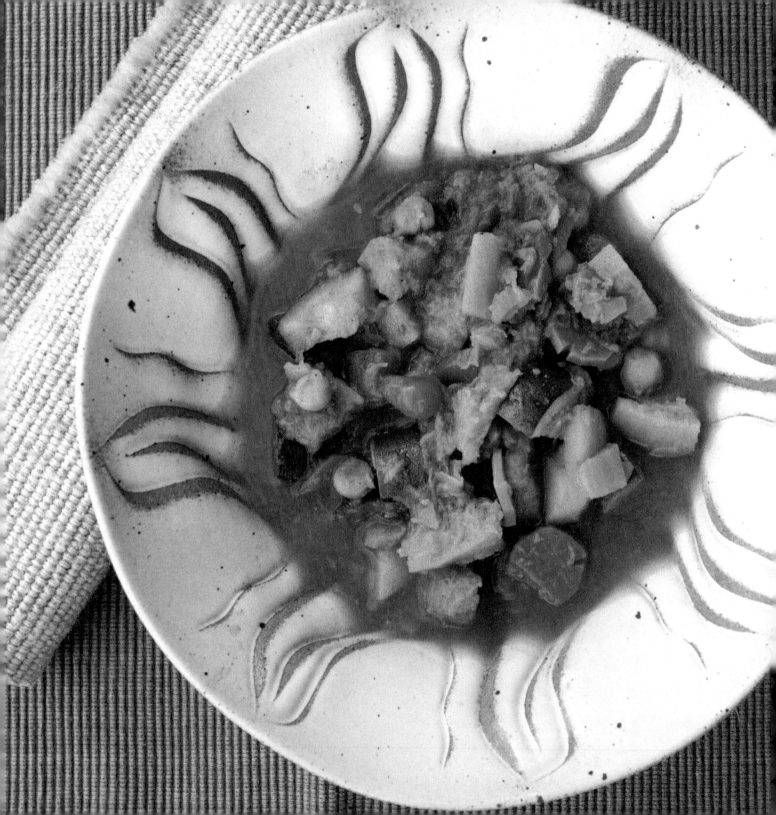

Moroccan Vegetable Stew

Ingredients:

1   large onion, chopped

1   tablespoon olive oil

2   teaspoons ground cinnamon

2   teaspoons ground cumin

1   teaspoon ground coriander

$1/2$ teaspoon cayenne pepper

$1/2$ teaspoon ground allspice

$1/4$ teaspoon salt

3   cups water

1   small butternut squash, peeled and cubed

2   medium potatoes, peeled and cubed

4   medium carrots, sliced

3   plum tomatoes, chopped

2   small zucchini, cut into 1-inch pieces

2   cups garbanzo beans or chickpeas

Servings: 8 servings (3 quarts)

Don't let the spices steer you away – absolutely delicious

In a large cooking pot, sauté onion in oil until tender. Add spices and salt; cook 1 minute longer.

Stir in the water, squash, potatoes, carrots and tomatoes. Bring to a boil.

Reduce heat; simmer, uncovered, for 15-20 minutes or until potatoes and squash are almost tender.

Add zucchini and chickpeas; return to a boil. Reduce heat; simmer, uncovered, for 5-8 minutes or until vegetables are tender.

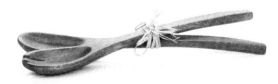

Nutty Veggie Burgers

Ingredients:

1/2 cup walnuts
2   cups cooked beans (lentils, garbanzos, pintos, black beans or a combination of all)
2   tablespoons tahini
1   tablespoon olive oil
1/2 cup diced onion
1/2 cup sliced mushrooms
1   teaspoon sea salt
1/2 teaspoon black pepper
1/2 cup sunflower seeds
1   cup millet, rice or other cooked grain

Servings: 4

Toast walnuts at 375 ° for 8-10 minutes. Let cool and chop finely.

Puree' beans and tahini until smooth, adding water as needed.

In a medium skillet, heat olive oil and sauté' onion, mushrooms, salt, and pepper until mushrooms are limp. Let cool.

Combine bean mixture with mushroom mixture in a medium mixing bowl. Mix well, and stir in walnuts and sunflower seeds. Add grains and use hands to mix until well blended. Chill for 1-2 hours.

Shape burger mixture into patties about 3-4 inches wide. Sauté', grill, or broil until done in center (about 5 minutes per side).

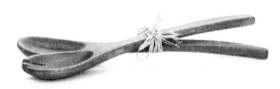

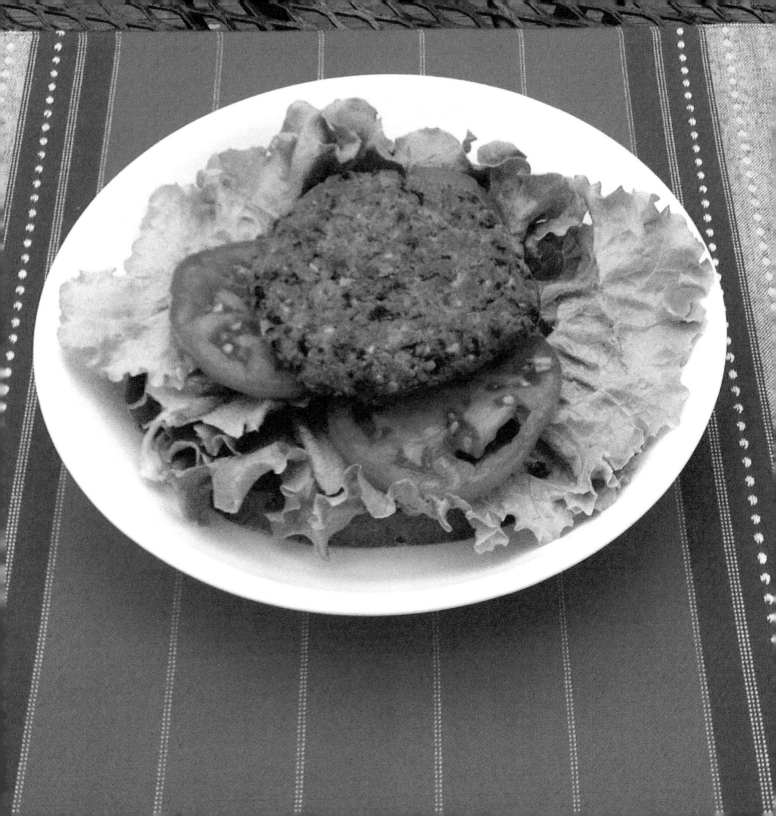

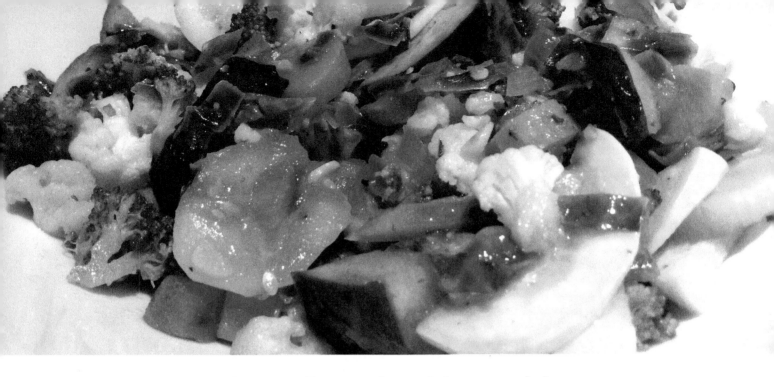

Oven Roasting Vegetables

The following recipes can be used with any vegetable such as asparagus, Brussels sprouts, eggplants, squash, zucchini, potatoes, carrots and even cucumbers. Liven up your meals, keep it simple and easy and most of make it flavorful. Be creative with different spices.

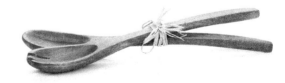

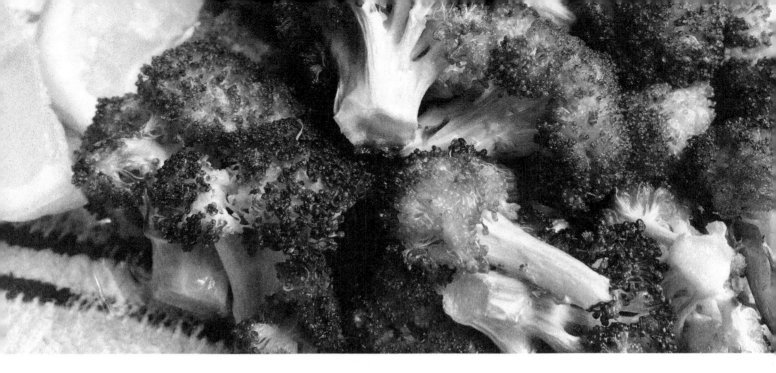

Oven-Roasted Broccoli

Ingredients:

2   cups broccoli florets

2   teaspoons olive oil

1   lemon

     Salt and pepper -- to taste

Serving Size: 4

Toss broccoli with olive oil. Lay florets in a single layer on a baking sheet. Add salt and pepper.

Roast at 400 ° for 12 -15 minutes or until crisp tender. Remove from oven and drizzle with fresh lemon juice. Serve immediately.

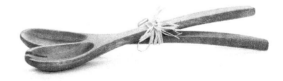

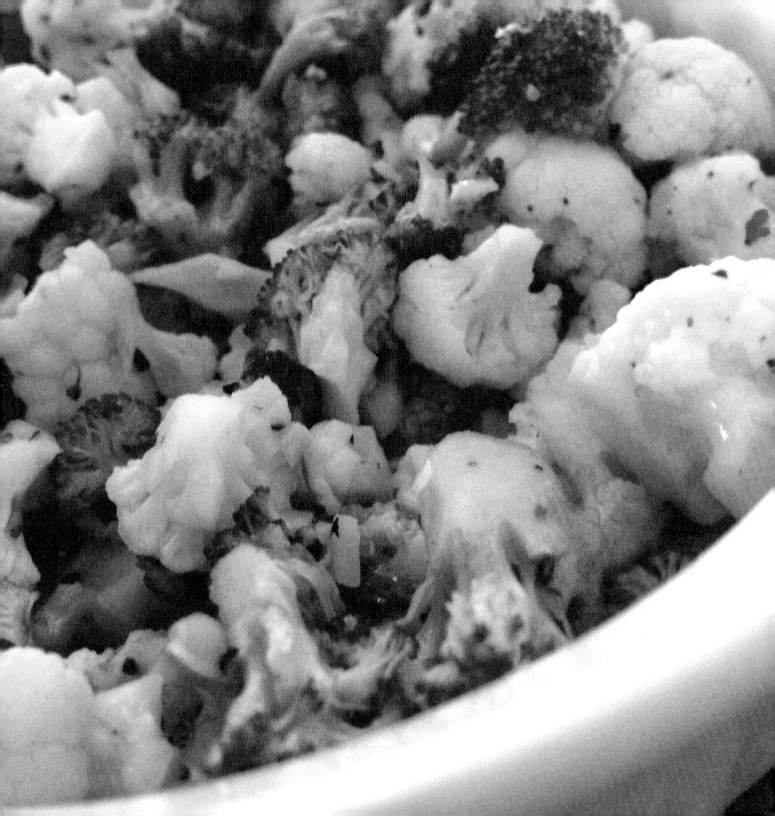

Oven Roasted Broccoli and Cauliflower

Ingredients:

6 cups small, bite-size fresh broccoli and cauliflower florets, mixed

2 to 3 tablespoons extra virgin olive oil

½ teaspoon salt

¼ teaspoon ground black pepper

2 garlic cloves, finely minced

¾ teaspoon crushed red pepper

Preheat to 425 °.

Toss broccoli and cauliflower in a large bowl with olive oil, salt and black pepper.

Add garlic and crushed red pepper; toss well to thoroughly coat all pieces.

Coat a shallow baking pan (10x15x1-inch jelly roll pan) with cooking spray and arrange vegetables in single layer.

Roast 10 to 15 minutes or until slightly tender and beginning to brown but not burn.

Stir all vegetables once during cooking time.

Serve immediately

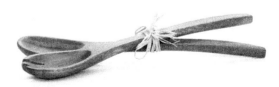

Peruvian Quinoa Stew

Ingredients:

- ½ cup uncooked quinoa
- 1 cup water
- 2 cups chopped onions
- 2 cloves garlic -- minced or pressed
- 1 tablespoon vegetable oil
- 1 stalk celery – sliced
- 1 carrot – cut on the diagonal into ¼-inch thick slices
- 1 bell pepper – cut into 1-inch pieces
- 1 cup zucchini – cubed
- 2 cups diced fresh or canned tomatoes – undrained
- 1 cup water or vegetable stock
- 2 teaspoons ground cumin
- ½ teaspoon chili powder
- 1 teaspoon ground coriander
- Pinch cayenne – to taste
- 1 teaspoon dried oregano
- Chopped fresh cilantro – for garnish

Serving Size: 4

Place quinoa and water in pot (covered) and cook covered on medium-low heat for about 15 minute until soft.

While the quinoa is cooking place the onions, garlic and vegetable oil in covered soup pot and sauté on medium heat for 5 minutes

Add celery and carrots to the soup pot and cook an additional 5 minutes, stirring often

Add the bell pepper, zucchini, tomatoes, and one cup water or vegetable stock to soup pot. Stir in cumin, chili powder, coriander, cayenne and oregano to soup pot simmer covered for 10 to 15 minutes until vegetables are tender.

Stir in cooked quinoa and salt to taste.

Top with grated cheese and optionally chopped cilantro

Serve immediately.

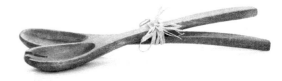

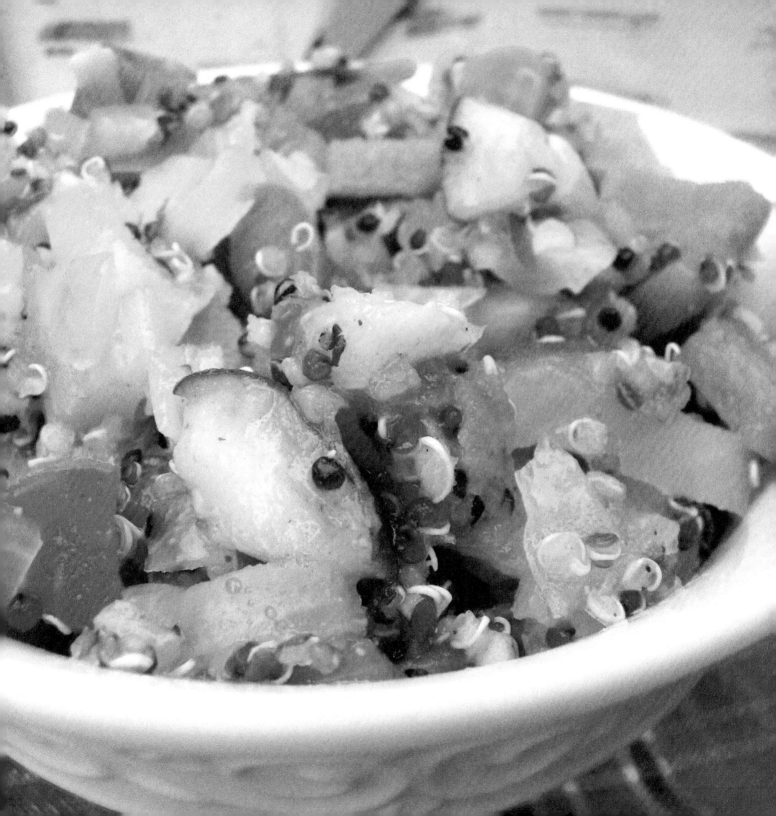

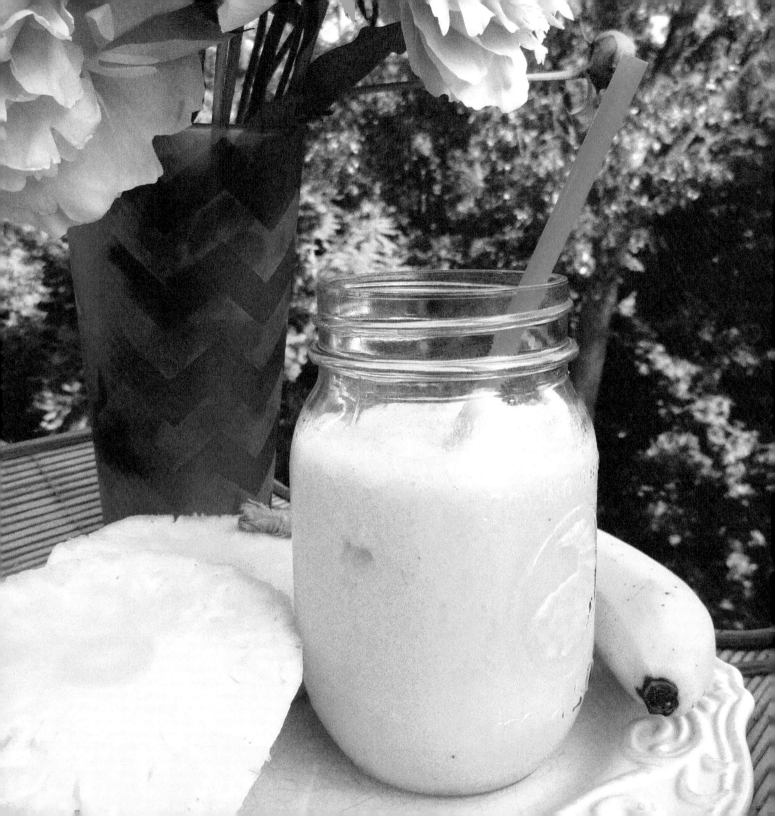

Pine-Orange-Banana Smoothie

Ingredients:

1	banana – sliced
½	cup pineapple – fresh, cut in bite size pieces
½	cup orange juice – freshly squeezed
2	teaspoons honey (omit for Daniel Fast)

Serving Size: 1

Put all ingredients in blender and process until smooth.

For a frozen smoothie, add ice cubes and process.

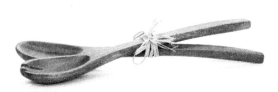

Popeye Burgers

Ingredients:

- 1   box frozen chopped spinach – thawed
- 1   large potato – grated
- 1   medium onion – finely chopped
- 1   tablespoon garlic powder
- 1   tablespoon dried minced onion
- ½   teaspoon paprika
- ½   cup tomato sauce
- ½   cup crushed whole wheat matzo
- ½   cup rolled oats
- ½   cup cornmeal
- 1   teaspoon seasoned salt
- 1   teaspoon Dijon mustard

Serving Size: 4

Blend all ingredients thoroughly in a large mixing bowl, adding a little more cornmeal if the mixture is too wet or a little water if the mixture is too dry.

Form into thin patties (the thinner the better) and fry in a lightly oiled nonstick pan over medium heat.

Uncooked patties may be frozen.

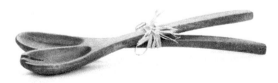

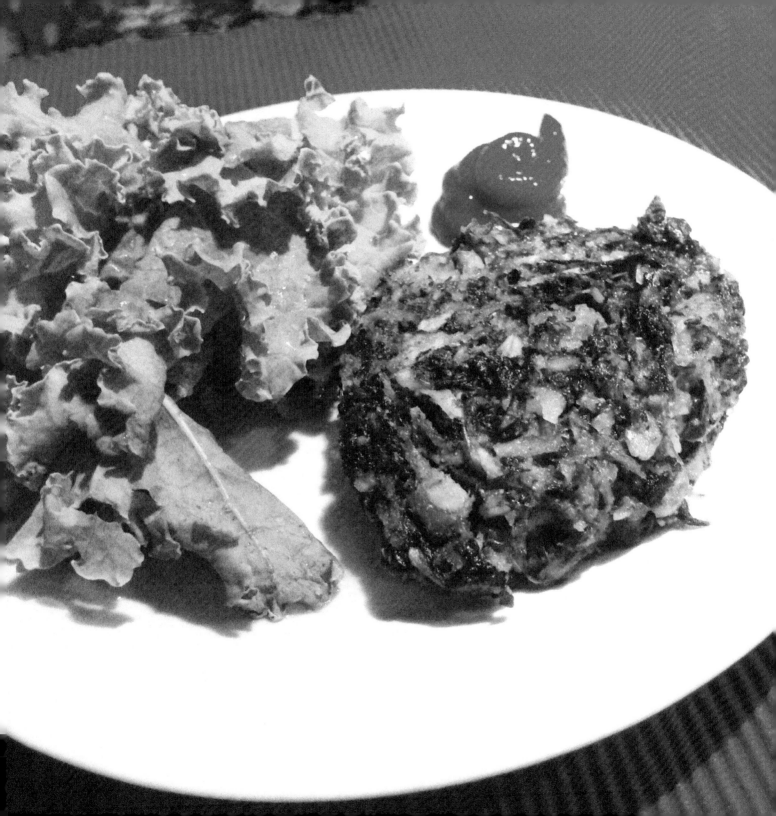

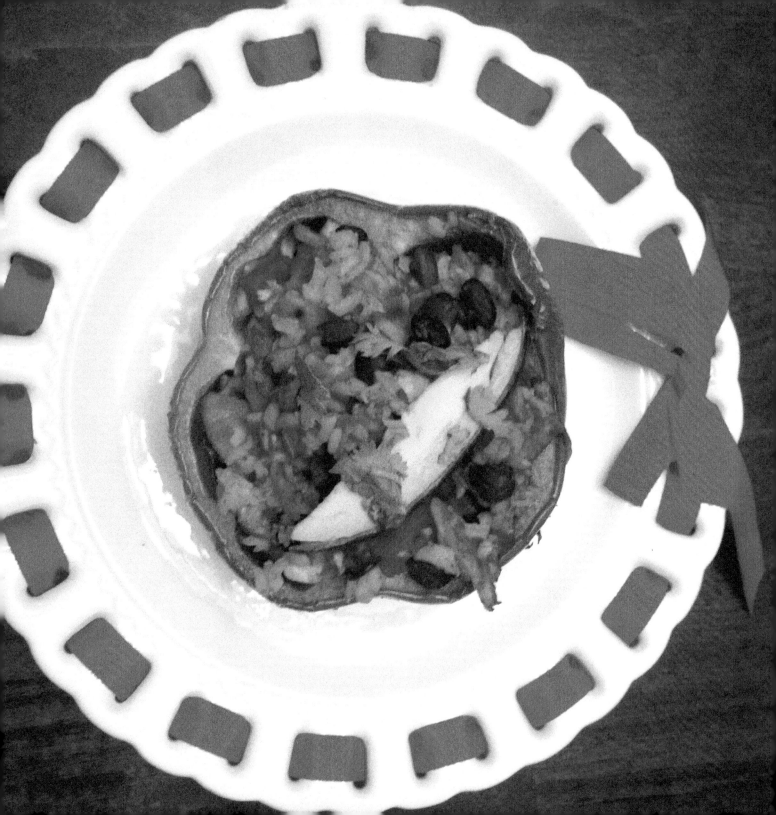

Savory Stuffed Peppers

Ingredients:

Olive Oil

1   cup chopped onions

1   tablespoons chili powder

½   teaspoon cumin

¼   teaspoon paprika

½   teaspoon salt

¼   teaspoon pepper

vteaspoon cayenne pepper

2 cups of cooked brown rice

½   cup shredded carrots

¾   cup chopped mushrooms

3-4 organic bell peppers, halved and seeds removed

2   cups black beans, cooked and drained

½   cup of organic frozen corn

2   cups – your favorite salsa

Toppings:

Fresh cilantro

Sliced avocado

Pre heat the oven to 400°. Lightly coat the peppers with olive oil and roast in a baking dish about 20-25 minutes just until cooked through. Remove the peppers from the oven and let cool for handling.

In a bowl mix all seasonings, onions, black beans, corn, carrots, mushrooms and rice. Add in the salsa and mix well.

Carefully spoon the rice mixture into each half of the bell peppers and place back on the baking dish. Cook the stuffed peppers for another 15-20 minutes or until the peppers are cooked all the way thru.

Remove from the oven and top with fresh cilantro and avocado slices just before serving.

*After the Daniel Fast this recipe is even better with ½ pound cooked ground turkey added to the rice mixture and then topped with your favorite cheese after cooking.

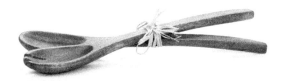

Spanish Paella

Ingredients:

½	cup long-grain brown rice
2	cups vegetable stock – or water
½	cup basmati rice
1	tablespoon olive oil
1	large yellow onion
2	cloves garlic – minced
1	medium red pepper – chopped
1	medium green pepper – chopped
½	cup fresh mushrooms – sliced
1½	cups eggplant – cubed
½	cup sliced black olives
1	teaspoon sea salt
½	teaspoon black pepper
½	teaspoon ground cumin
½	teaspoon saffron
1	pound tomatoes – coarsely chopped

Serving Size: 4

Combine brown rice and stock in large saucepan. Bring to a boil, and then reduce to simmer and cook, covered, about 10 minutes. Add basmati rice and cook for an additional 30 minutes.

Preheat oven to 400 °.

While rice is cooking, heat oil in a large, oven-proof skillet and add chopped onion, garlic, red pepper, green pepper, saffron, mushrooms, eggplant, olives, salt, pepper and cumin. Sauté until peppers are tender (about 5 minutes).

Stir tomatoes and rice mixture into vegetables and bake in 400 degree oven for about 10 minutes or until heated through and bubbly.

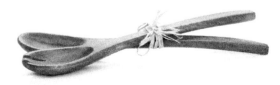

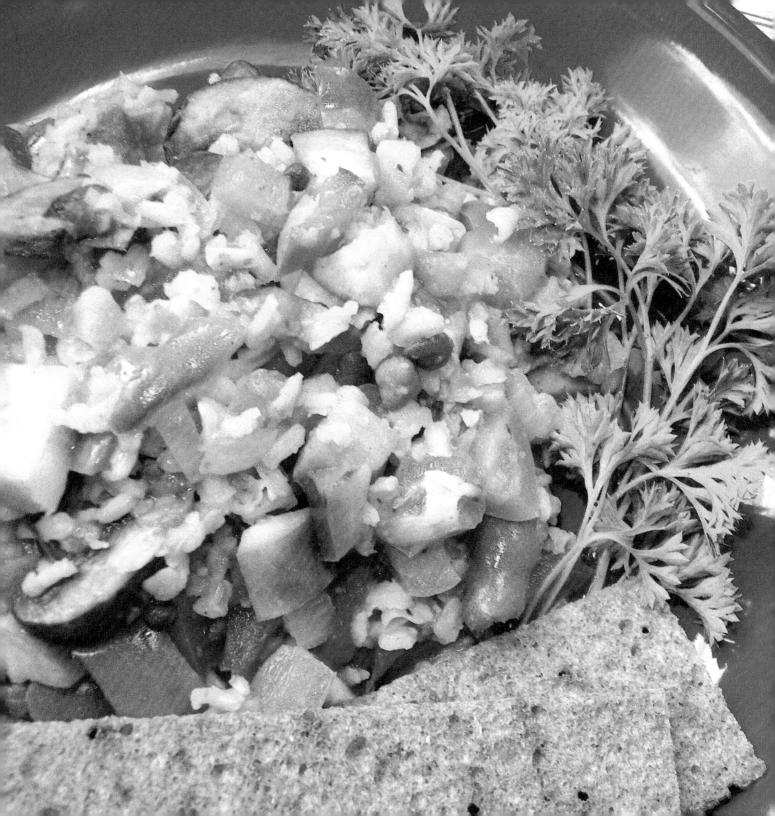

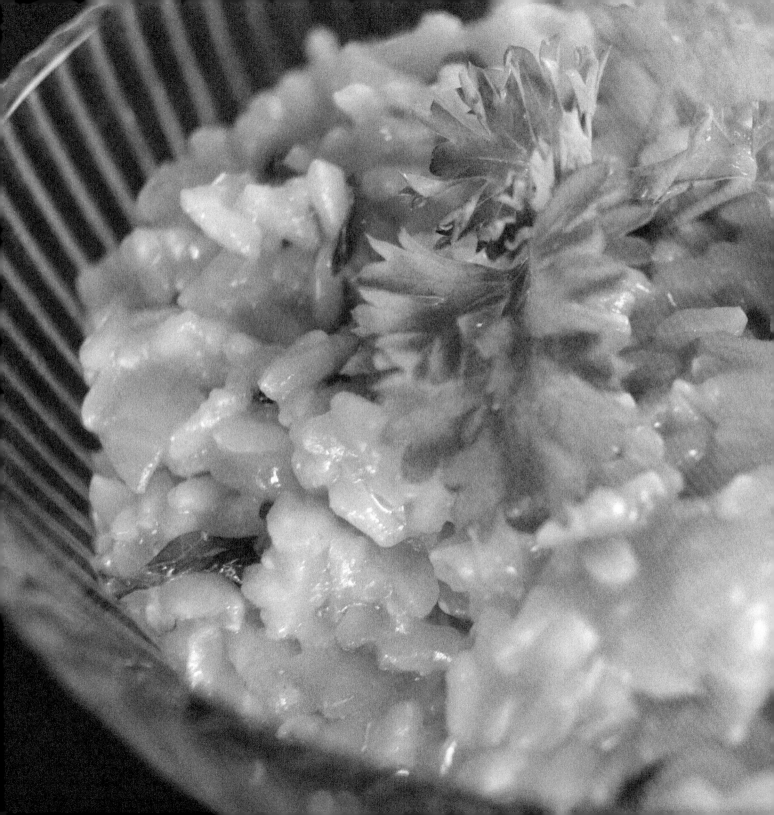

Sweet Brown Rice with Spicy Sauce

Ingredients:

1	teaspoon olive oil
1	yellow onion
3	cloves garlic – minced
2	tablespoons minced fresh ginger
1/3	cup water
2	tablespoons Braggs Liquid Aminos
1/2	teaspoon chili sauce
2	teaspoons sesame oil
4	tablespoons chopped fresh cilantro
4	cups cooked short grain brown rice

Serving Size: 4

Heat olive oil in large skillet over medium high heat; add onion, garlic and gingerroot and sauté' for about 2 minutes or until onion softens.

Add water, Liquid Aminos, chili sauce, sesame oil and half of the cilantro; stir until well blended and then reduce heat to medium.

Add brown rice and cover pan; continue to cook until rice absorbs most of the liquid and all ingredients are well heated, 5-7 minutes.

Transfer to serving bowl, garnish with remaining cilantro.

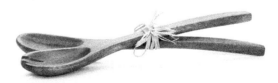

Sweet Potato Pie

Ingredients:

- 8   peeled sweet potatoes – cooked, cooled and smashed
- 3   cups broccoli – fresh and chopped
- 2   cups collard greens – chopped
- 2   cups cauliflower – fresh or frozen chopped
- 1/2   pound mushrooms – sliced
- 6   garlic cloves – minced
- 1   red pepper – seeded and chopped
- 2 1/2   cups vegetable broth
- 3   teaspoons chili powder
- 3   tablespoons tomato paste
- 2   teaspoons Bragg Liquid Amino
- 2   tablespoons raw nut butter
- 3   cups red beans – cooked
- 1/2   cup pecans – chopped

Servings: 8

Recipe: *The Antioxidant Diet;* Robin Jeep and Dr. Couey

In a large pot, combine broccoli, collard greens, cauliflower, mushrooms and bell peppers in broth and simmer covered for 15 minutes. Add chili powder, tomato paste and Bragg's Liquid Aminos; cook until almost tender (about 10 minutes).

Mix in nut butter and beans and spread the mixture in baking dish. Spread sweet potatoes over the top and sprinkle with a little additional chili powder and chopped pecans.

Bake 20-30 minutes until hot and pecans are light brown, about 20 minutes.

This dish can be prepared ahead and frozen, baked or unbaked.

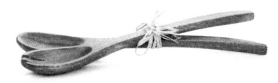

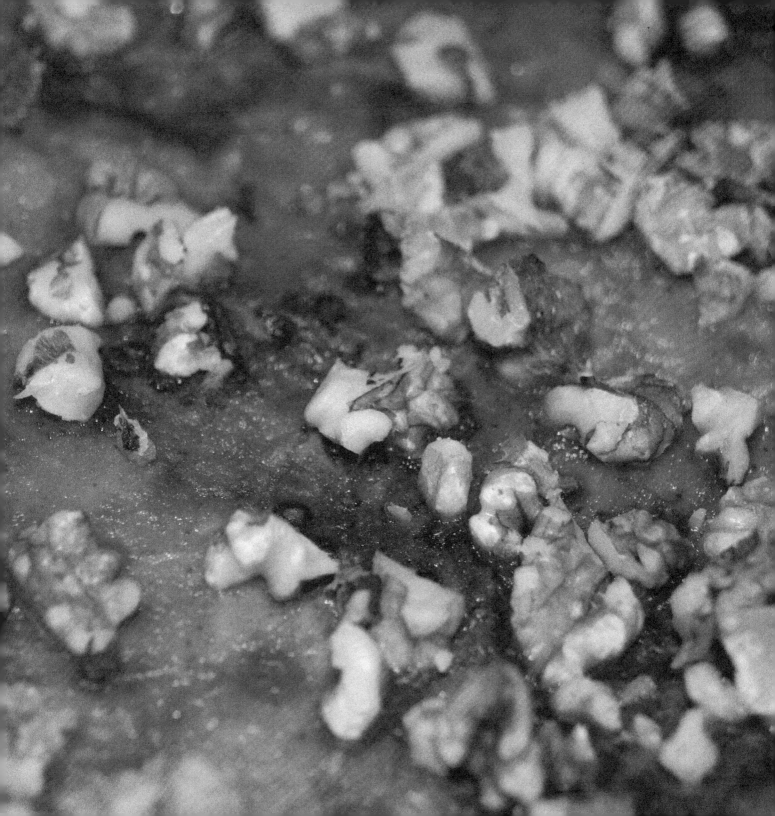

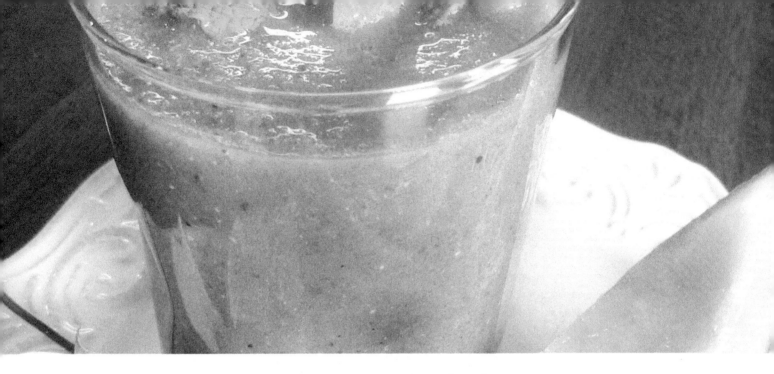

Surprise Delight

Ingredients:

1   cup unsweetened pineapple juice

1   cup water

1   cup frozen pineapple chunks

1   cup cubed cantaloupe

1   raw carrot

4   kale leaves, stripped from stems

1   kiwi, peeled and sliced

1   tablespoon freshly ground flaxseed

Servings: 2

Recipe: *The Antioxidant Diet;* Robin Jeep and Dr. Couey

Combine in a blender and blend until smooth.

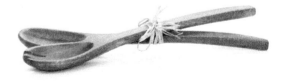

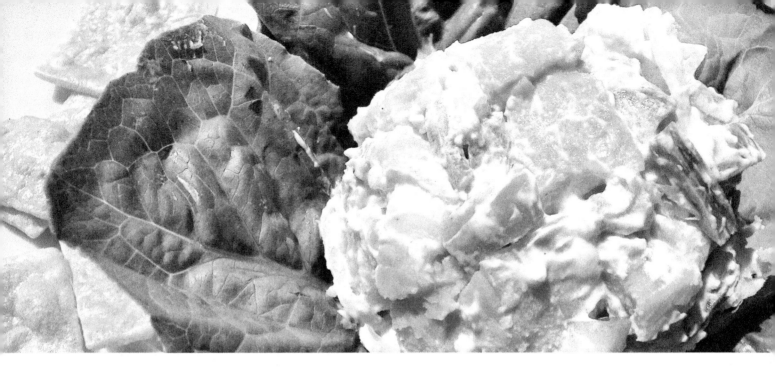

Sweet Potato Salad

Ingredients:

3   pounds sweet potatoes, cooked, peeled and cubed

1   cup green pepper, chopped

½   cup onion, finely

1½ teaspoon salt

¼   teaspoon pepper

1½ cups unflavored yogurt
    Dash pepper

Servings: 4-5

In a large bowl, combine the first five ingredients. Stir in yogurt and pepper sauce. Cover and refrigerate for at least 1 hour before serving. Yield: 10 servings.

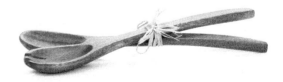

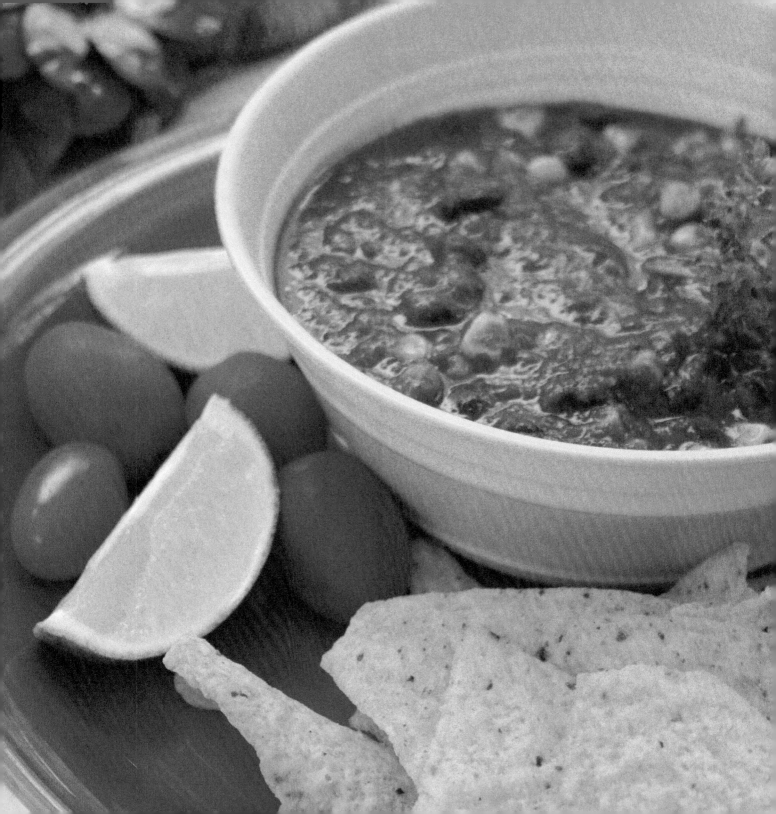

Tex Mex Chili

Ingredients:

2	tablespoons olive oil
1½	cups chopped onions
6	garlic cloves, minced
2	tablespoons jalapeno peppers, rinsed and squeezed
1	tablespoon cumin
2	teaspoons oregano
½	teaspoon cinnamon
1	garlic clove, minced
1	teaspoon ground coriander
1	tablespoon chili powder
½	teaspoon black pepper
½	teaspoon salt, to taste
2	cups black beans, cooked
2	cups stewed tomatoes
2	cups organic sweet corn
1	ounce baker's chocolate or 1/8 cup dark chocolate pieces
1	tablespoon lime juice
1	tablespoon Bragg's Liquid Aminos

Sauté onions and garlic in olive oil until soft and starting to caramelize.

Add spices, jalapenos and stewed tomatoes, simmer for 5 minutes.

Using an immersion blender, grind this mixture until smooth (or put in blender).

Add beans, corn, chocolate, lime juice and liquid aminos.

Simmer for 20 minutes.

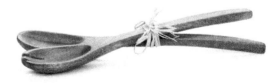

Three-Bean Indian Dal

Ingredients:

2	tablespoons olive oil
1	medium red onion – diced
½	cup celery – sliced thin
4	cloves garlic – minced or pressed
1	small green pepper – diced
1	teaspoon sea salt
½	teaspoon white pepper
1	tablespoon celery seed
1	tablespoon ground cumin
2	teaspoons coriander
2	tablespoons fresh ginger –- grated
2	large tomatoes
3	cups water
1	cup cooked lentils
1	cup black beans, cooked
1	cup garbanzo beans
¼	cup cilantro – chopped

Serving Size: 6

Heat oil in large soup pot and sauté onion, celery, garlic, green pepper, salt and white pepper until green pepper is tender. Add celery seed, ground cumin, coriander, and ginger and sauté 3 minutes longer.

Core tomatoes and dice. Add to onion and pepper mixture, and sauté until tomatoes are soft and juicy.

Add water, lentils, black beans, garbanzo beans and cilantro to soup pot and simmer, covered for 10-15 minutes. Serve hot, garnished with cilantro.

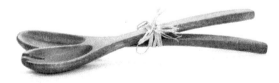

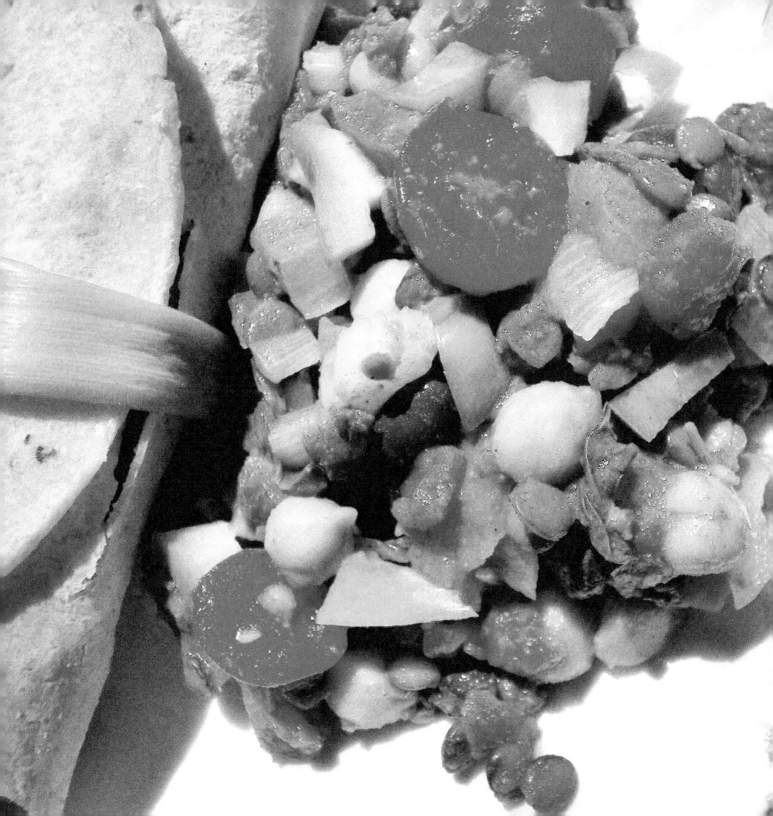

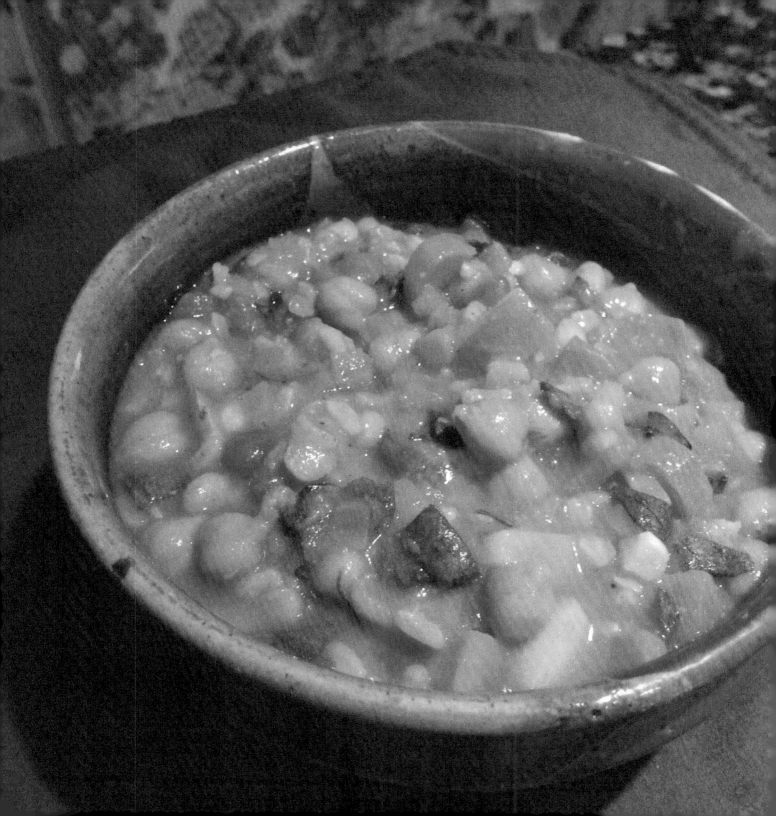

Three Bean Soup

Ingredients:

1   tablespoon olive oil
1   cup chopped onion
3   cloves garlic, minced
1   teaspoon dried rosemary leaves
1/4   teaspoon dried thyme leaves
2   bay leaves
1   whole clove
1/4   teaspoon pepper
5   cups vegetable broth
1½   cups cooked baby lima beans (sub. navy beans)
1½   cups cooked chickpeas
1½   cups cooked red beans
3   tablespoons tomato paste
1½   cups cooked barley or rice
1   large potato, unpeeled, cut into ½-inch pieces
1   cup sliced carrots
1   cup packed chopped spinach leaves

Servings: 6

Heat oil in large soup pot over medium heat; sauté onions, and garlic for 2-3 minutes or until onions are tender.

Add vegetable broth, beans, spices and tomato paste to pot; heat to boiling, stirring to prevent sticking.

Reduce heat and simmer, uncovered, for 10-15 minutes.

Add barley, potato, carrots, and spinach and simmer 10 more minutes until all ingredients are well heated.

Discard bay leaves and clove before serving.

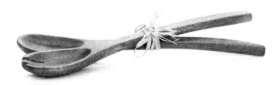

Toasted Almond Granola

Ingredients:

4   cups old fashioned oats
1   cup slivered raw almonds
1   cup whole raw almonds
1/2   cup unsweetened shredded coconut
1   teaspoon ground cinnamon
1/2   teaspoon salt
3   tablespoons butter
1/4   cup olive oil
1/4   cup honey
1/2   cup sucanat – any variety
1   teaspoon pure vanilla extract

This recipe uses honey and sucanat so you may opt to save it for after the fast. It is delicious so make it an addition to your favorites.

Servings: 8 cups

Place a rack in the upper third and middle of the oven and preheat to 325 ° F. Line one large or two small baking sheets with parchment paper and set aside.

Stir together oats, whole almonds, slivered almonds, unsweetened coconut cinnamon and salt. Set aside.

In a medium saucepan, melt together butter, oil, honey and sucanat until the sucanat is dissolved and the mixture begins to boil. Carefully stir together until well mixed. Add the vanilla extract. Pour the warm mixture over the oat and almond mixture and toss together with a wooden spoon, ensuring that all of the oat mixture gets moistened by the honey and oil mixture.

Spread mixture onto prepared baking sheet(s) and bake for about 25 to 30 minutes, Stir the mixture twice during baking. Remove from the oven, let cool and store in an airtight container for up to two weeks.

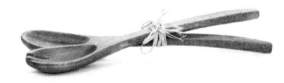

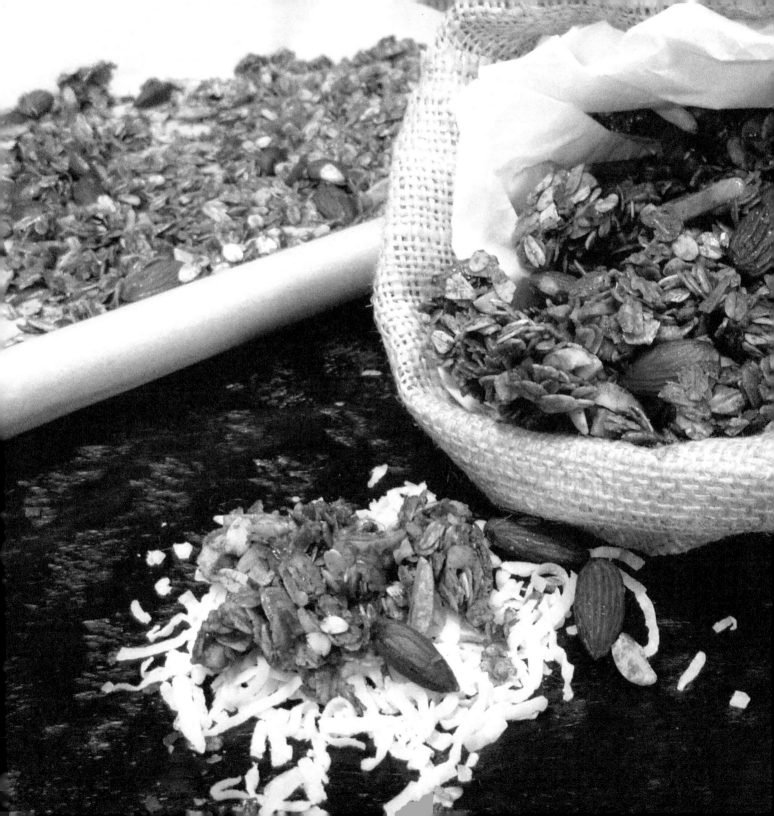

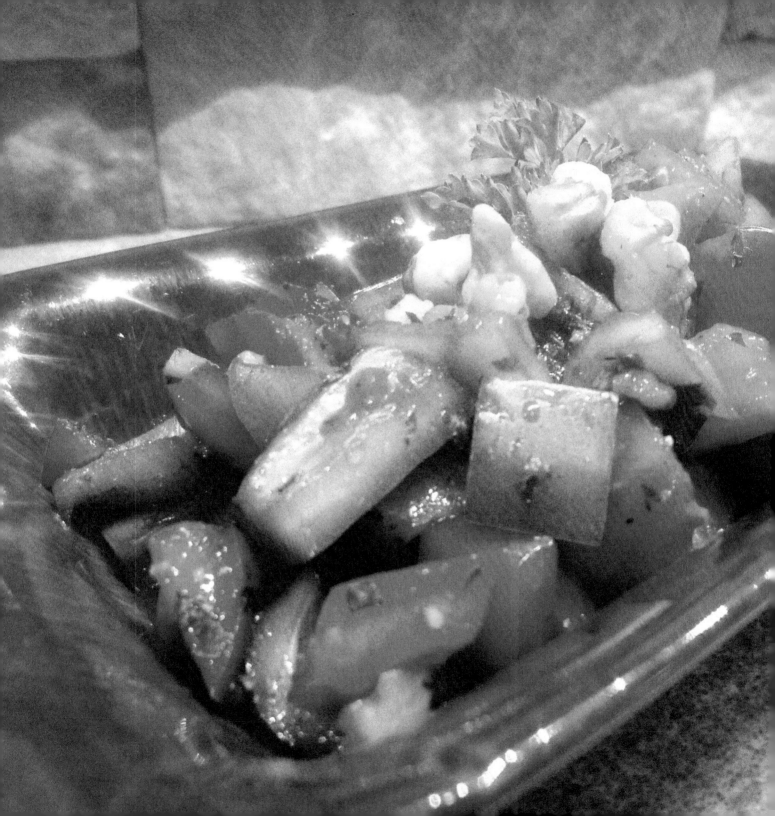

Tomato Walnut Salad

Ingredients:

3   tomatoes, chopped

2   green bell peppers, seeded and
chopped

$^1/_2$ cup chopped walnuts

$^1/_4$ cup fresh parsley leaves, chopped
finely

$1^1/_2$ tablespoons molasses
extra-virgin olive oil to taste
salt and pepper to taste

In a salad bowl toss together the tomatoes, peppers, walnuts, parsley, molasses, olive oil and salt and pepper to taste.

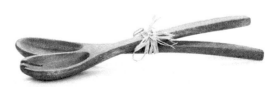

Turkish Salad

Ingredients:

1 head green leaf lettuce – torn into bite sized pieces
1 green bell pepper – cut in thin strips
1 red bell pepper – cut in thin strips
1/2 cucumber – seeded and sliced
1 red onion – slice into half rings
4 tomatoes – diced
1 cup pitted black olives

Dressing:

3 tablespoons extra virgin olive oil
3 tablespoons lemon juice
1 clove garlic – minced
1 tablespoon fresh Italian parsley – finely chopped
1 tablespoon fresh mint – finely chopped
Salt and pepper – to taste

Serving Size: 4

Place lettuce, peppers, cucumber and tomatoes and onion in large serving bowl.

Whisk together dressing ingredients in separate bowl.

Just before serving, whisk dressing again and pour over salad vegetable and gently toss to coat.

Add olives and gently toss again. Serve

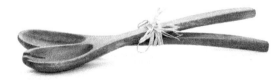

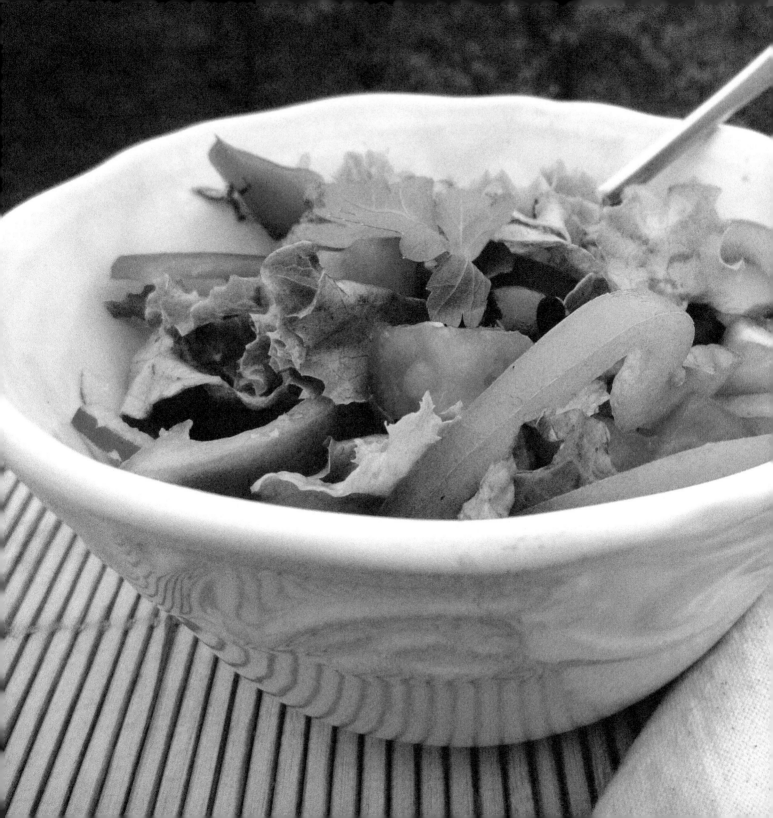

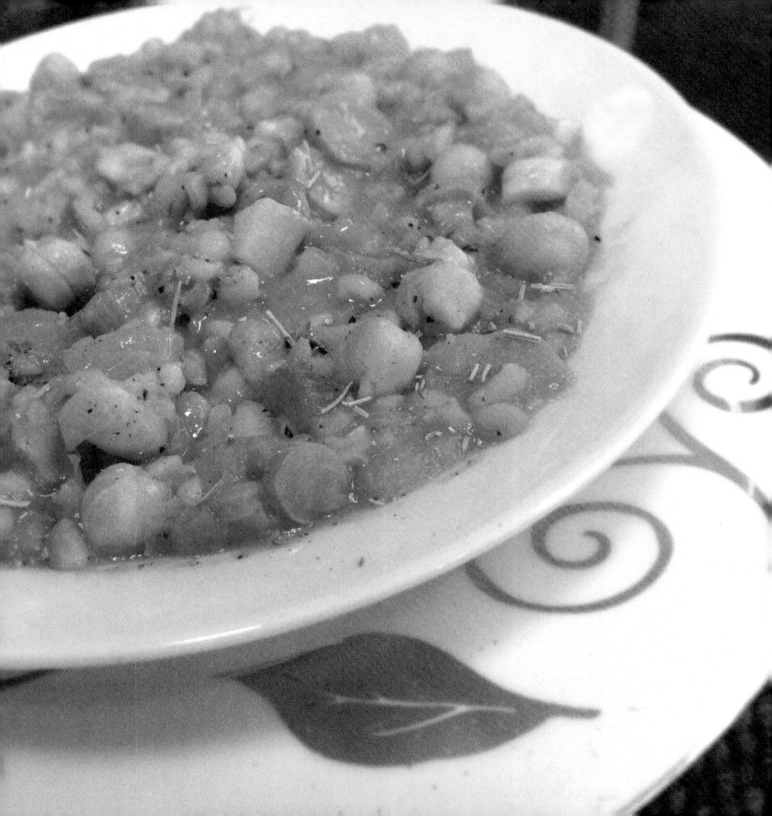

Tuscan Villa Bean Soup

Ingredients:

1	tablespoon olive oil
1	cup chopped onion
1/2	cup finely chopped celery – optional
3	cloves garlic – minced
1	tablespoon whole wheat flour
1	teaspoon dried rosemary leaves – crushed
1/4	teaspoon dried thyme leaves – crushed
2	bay leaves – whole
1	clove – whole
1/4	teaspoon pepper
5	cups vegetable broth
1 1/2	cups white beans, cooked and drained
1 1/2	cups chickpeas, cooked and drained
1/3	cup organic catsup
1 1/2	cups cooked barley or brown rice
1	large red or white potato, cut into small pieces
1	cup sliced carrots

Heat oil in large soup pot over medium heat and sauté onions, celery and garlic for 2-3 minutes or until onions are tender.

Stir in flour and seasonings.

Add vegetable broth, beans and catsup to onions. Heat to boiling, stirring to prevent sticking.

Reduce heat and simmer, uncovered for 10-15 minutes.

Add barley (or rice), potato, and carrots; simmer 10 more minutes until all ingredients are tender and heated.

Discard bay leaves and clove (if you can find it) before serving.

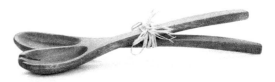

Tuscan White Bean Salad

4 cups Cannelloni beans or other white beans – drained

2 cloves fresh garlic – peeled and minced

1 cup fresh plum tomatoes – coarsely chopped

½ cup red onion – coarsely chopped

½ cup Italian parsley – chopped

½ cup sage, oregano or basil (or combination) – fresh, finely chopped

¼ cup red wine vinegar – May need up to ½ cup

Few drops balsamic vinegar (optional)

Extra virgin olive oil – to drizzle over salad

Salt and pepper – to taste

6 cups fresh baby spinach – washed, stems removed

Serving Size: 6

In a medium bowl, combine the first 6 ingredients

Add wine vinegar and balsamic vinegar and toss gently to mix but not break up beans.

Drizzle a small amount of olive oil over bean mixture and toss lightly.

Season with salt and freshly ground black pepper to taste.

May serve plain or on a bed of spinach, at room temperature or chilled, as desired.

Accompany with toasted slices of baguette drizzled with olive oil.
Comments: Tuscan bean salad is very common on antipasto menus and tables in Tuscany. The salad may be served at room temperature or chilled.

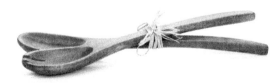

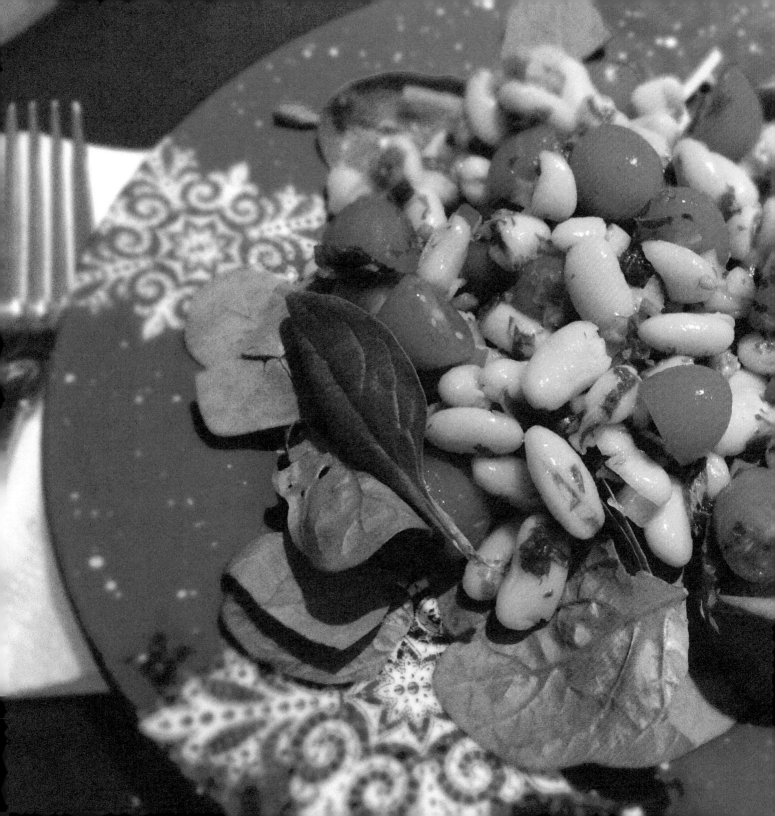

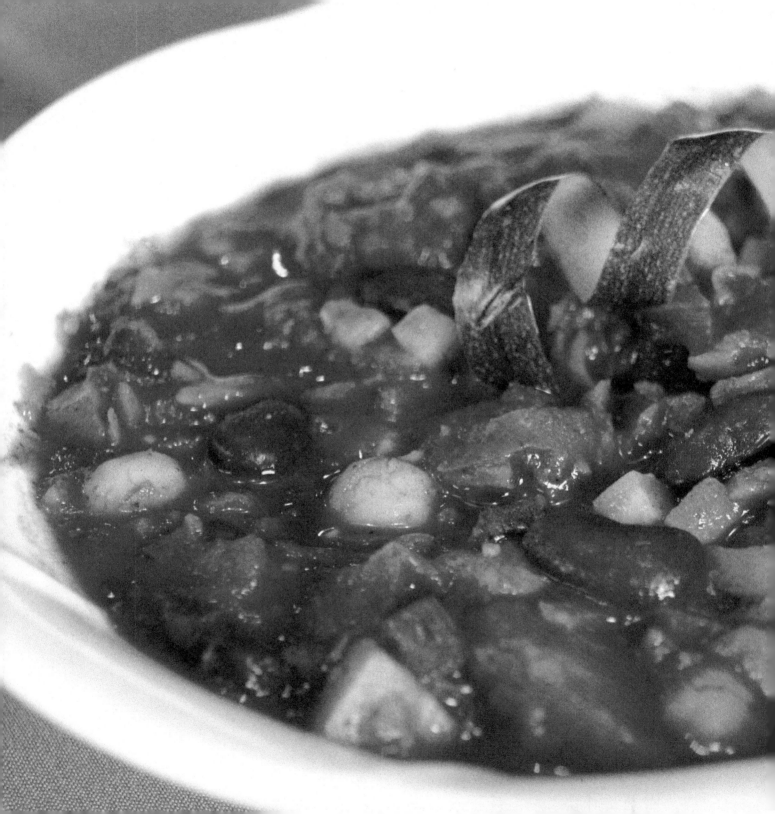

Vegetarian Chili

Ingredients:

½   cup chopped onion

⅓   cup chopped green bell pepper

1⅓ cloves garlic – minced

2   tablespoons olive oil

1⅓ tablespoons chili powder

⅓   teaspoon oregano

⅓   teaspoon cumin

⅓   teaspoon ground black pepper

1⅓ cups zucchini – finely chopped

⅔   cup carrots – shredded

3   cups diced tomatoes with juice

2   cups kidney beans – 2- 15½ oz. cans

1   cup garbanzo beans – 1- 15½ oz. can

Serving Size: 8

In large pot, sauté onions, peppers, and garlic in olive oil until soft.

Mix in chili powder, oregano, cumin, black pepper. Stir in zucchini and carrots. Cook for 1 hour over low heat, stirring occasionally. Add ½ to one cup of water if necessary.

Stir in tomatoes, kidney beans and chick peas. Bring to a boil. Reduce heat and simmer 30-45 minutes or until thick.

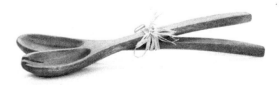

Vegetable Fried Rice

Ingredients:

1   cup cooked brown rice

2   eggs, lightly beaten – omit while on Daniel Fast

2   teaspoons organic canola oil (sub. Coconut or olive oil)

6   ounces asparagus spears, trimmed and cut into 1-inch pieces (about ½ bunch)

1   medium red bell pepper, thinly sliced into 1-inch pieces

4   scallions, cut into 1-inch pieces – or green onions

1   clove garlic, minced

1   tablespoon minced fresh ginger

4   teaspoons Bragg's Liquid Aminos

2   tablespoons rice vinegar

1   teaspoon toasted sesame oil

    Hot red pepper sauce, to taste

Coat a large nonstick wok or skillet with cooking spray and turn on medium heat. Pour in eggs and cook, stirring gently, until just set, 30 seconds to 1 minute. Transfer to a small bowl.

Heat oil in the pan over medium-high; add asparagus and cook, stirring, for 2 minutes. Add bell pepper, scallions, garlic and ginger; cook, stirring, until the vegetables are just tender, about 2 minutes.

Add the cooked rice, liquid aminos and vinegar to the pan; cook until the liquid is absorbed, 30 seconds to 1 minute.

Fold in the cooked eggs. Remove from the heat; stir in sesame oil and hot sauce.

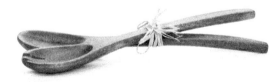

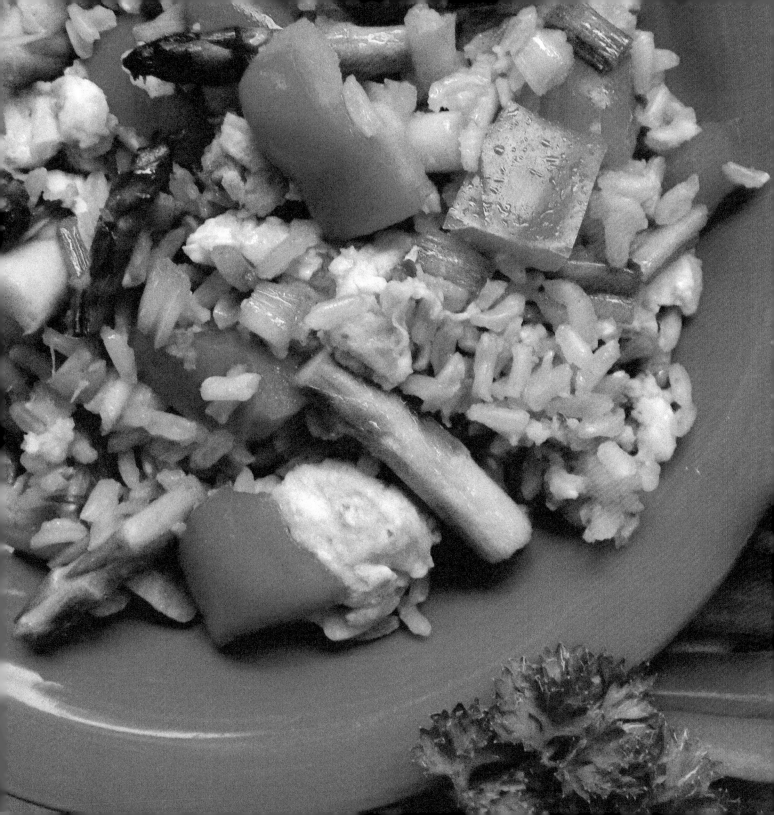

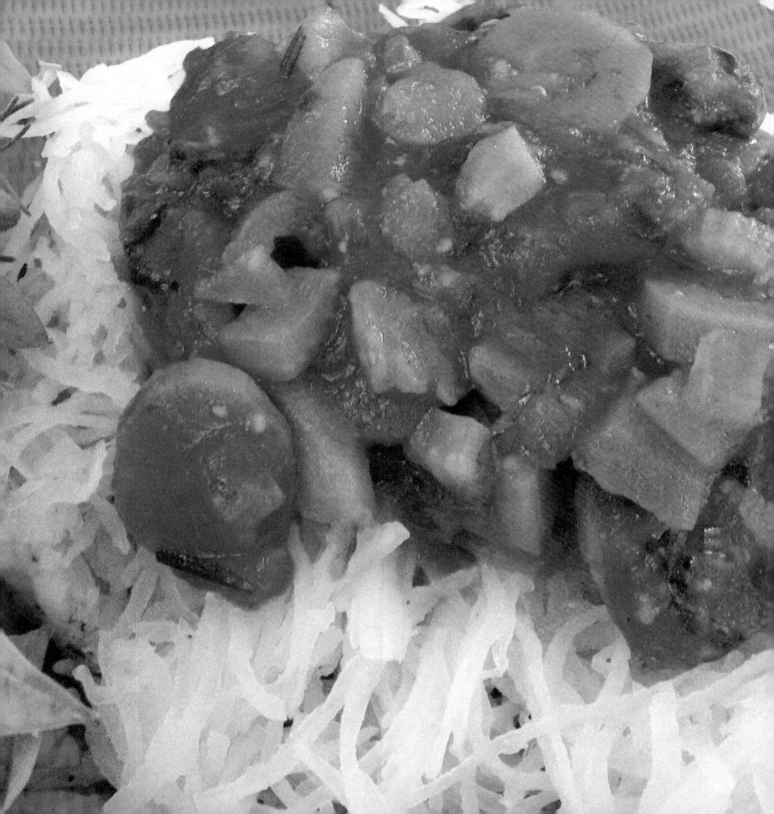

Veggie Medley Tomato Sauce

Ingredients:

2	tablespoons olive oil
1	clove garlic – minced
1	small onion – minced
1	cup chopped mushrooms
½	cup carrots – chopped
1	cup green pepper – chopped
½	cup celery – chopped
1	teaspoon black pepper
½	teaspoon salt
2	pounds Roma tomato – peeled and chopped
⅓	cup tomato paste
¼	cup fresh basil – finely chopped
2	tablespoons fresh oregano – chopped
2	tablespoons fresh thyme – chopped
2	tablespoons fresh rosemary – chopped

Serving Size: 8

Heat oil in large saucepan and sauté garlic until fragrant. Add minced onion, mushrooms, carrots, green peppers, celery, black pepper and salt. Cook just until carrots are tender.

Stir in tomatoes tomato paste and herbs, and simmer about 20 minutes. Serve hot over whole wheat pasta, spaghetti squash, or brown rice.

"Lots of fresh herbs and vegetables combine with ripe tomatoes to make this a hearty, low-fat sauce that complements almost any dish."

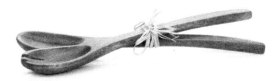

Vegetable Pizza

2 cups broccoli – chopped

1 large red bell pepper – seeded, chopped

1 cup mushrooms – sliced

1 garlic clove – minced

½ teaspoon Bragg Liquid Amino

1 tablespoons balsamic vinegar

1 teaspoon seasoning

½ cup pasta sauce

2 Ezekiel Sprouted Grain Tortillas

4 ounces soy or rice cheese – grated

5 ounces fresh spinach

Servings: 2

Recipe: *The Antioxidant Diet;* Robin Jeep & Dr. Couey

Preheat oven to 350 °. In a large bowl, toss broccoli, bell peppers and mushrooms with garlic, Bragg, vinegar and seasoning mix.

Roast vegetables on a lightly oiled cookie sheet, turning occasionally and mounding to keep from drying out, for 30 minutes.

Remove vegetables when done and preheat oven to 450 °. Spread a thin layer of pasta sauce on tortilla, sprinkle cheese and distribute roasted vegetables and spinach.

Bake on a cookie sheet for approximately 7 minutes or until cheese is melted and tortilla browns around edges.

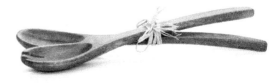

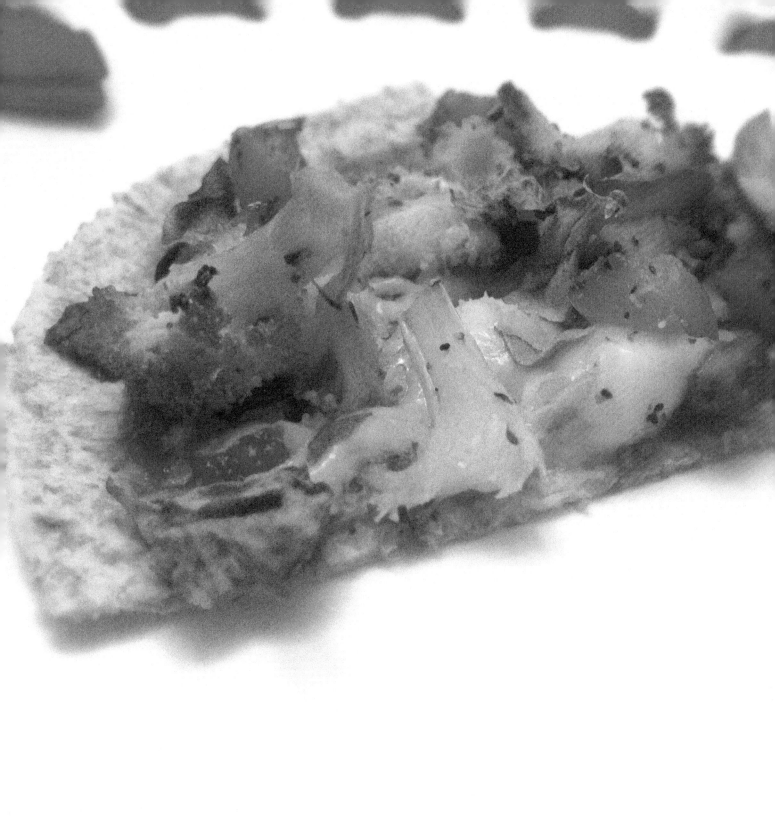

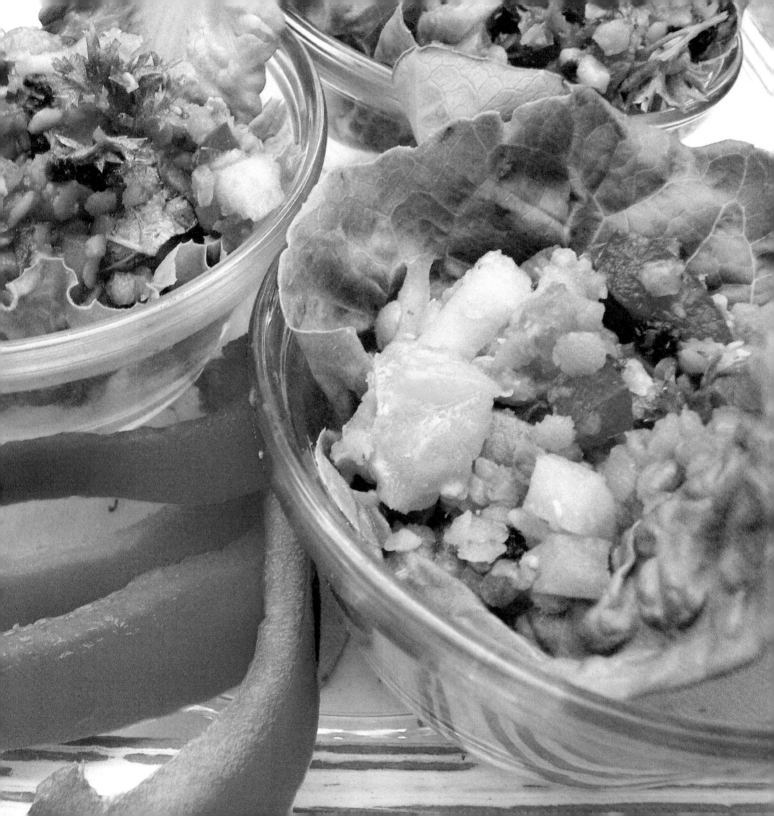

Veggie Wraps

Ingredients:

1   cup cooked lentils

½   cup celery – chopped

1   orange – peeled, sectioned and seeded

1   garlic clove – minced

½   tablespoon balsamic vinegar

3   teaspoons olive oil

1   tablespoon dried currants

¼   cup red pepper – chopped

1   tablespoon parsley - chopped

1   tablespoon mint – chopped

1   teaspoon Bragg Liquid Aminos

¼   cup walnuts – chopped

12 large leaf lettuce leaves

Servings: 4

Recipe: *The Antioxidant Diet;* Robin Jeep & Dr. Couey

Combine all ingredients except for lettuce leaves. Spread mixture on each lettuce leaf and roll.

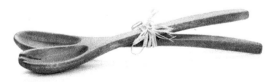

White Bean Dip

Ingredients:

3/4   cup dried white beans

1/4   cup bean cooking liquid

2   medium cloves garlic, peeled and
      minced

2   tablespoons chopped fresh dill

2   tablespoons chopped fresh mint

1   tablespoon chopped fresh flat-leaf
      parsley

1   tablespoon olive oil

2   teaspoons fresh lemon juice

1/4   teaspoon salt
      Red pepper powder – pinch to taste
      Additional olive oil and fresh herbs,
      for garnish

Soak the beans overnight in cold water. In the morning drain, reserving ¼ cup liquid.

Put the beans along with the reserved liquid in a blender or food processor, and blend with the garlic, dill, mint, parsley, olive oil, lemon juice, salt, and red pepper powder. Add more oil or bean liquid if needed. Puree until smooth.

Taste, and adjust for seasoning, adding more salt or olive oil if desired.

Garnish with a generous drizzle of olive oil and a scattering of fresh chopped herbs.

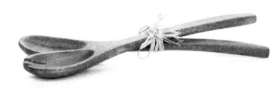

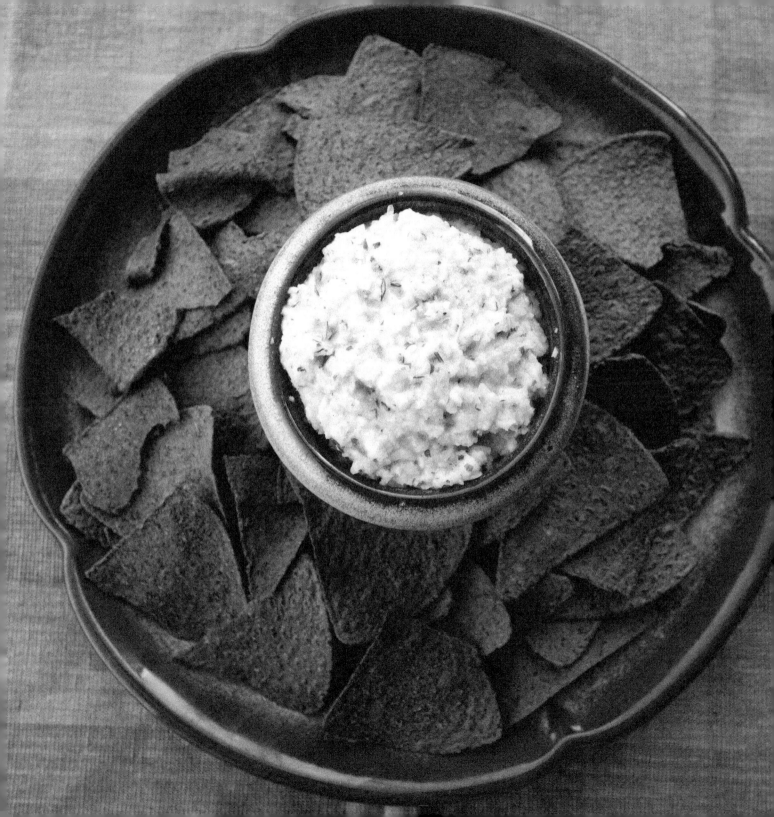

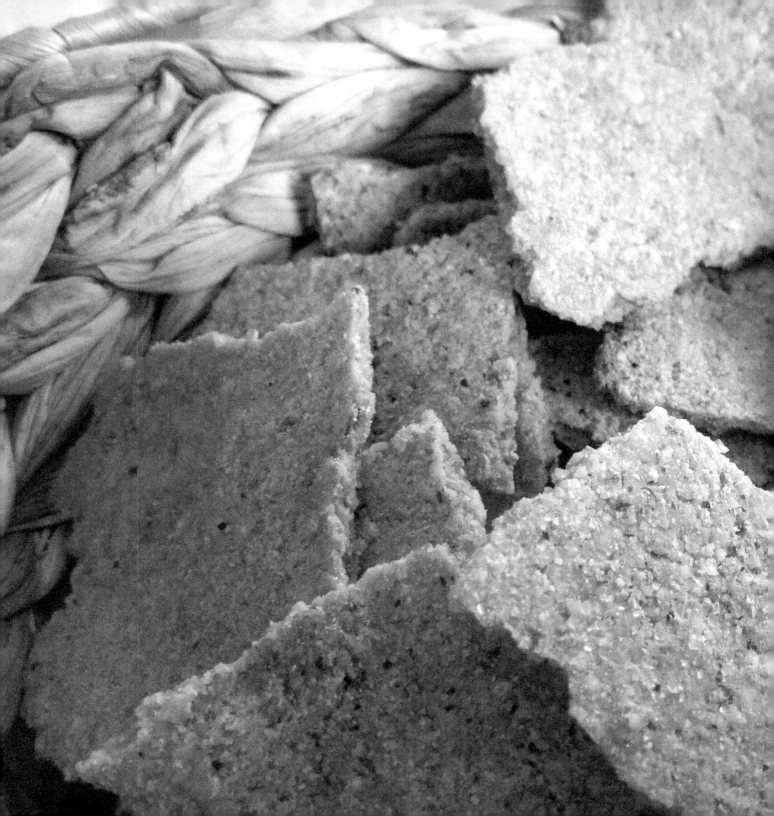

Whole Grain Crackers

Ingredients:

3/4 cup whole wheat flour

1/2 cup 7-grain Cereal

1/2 teaspoon salt

2 tablespoons olive oil

1/4 cup water

1 teaspoon seasoning of choice – chili powder, dried herbs, etc. – optional

Serving Size: 8

Preheat oven to 400°.

In a large bowl combine flour, cereal and salt. Add olive oil and water. Using a large rubber spatula or wooden spoon, stir vigorously until dough comes together and forms a ball. If it's too sticky to handle add flour - no more than a tablespoon at a time.

Dust the work surface with whole wheat flour and roll the dough out to 1/8 inch thickness, it should be very thin! Gently slide the dough onto a piece of parchment paper or silicone baking mat and place on a cookie sheet or flip a sheet pan upside down and slide the parchment with the dough on to the pan.

Bake at 400° for 12-15 minutes or until light brown. Cool for 10-15 minutes on a wire rack. Break into pieces about the size of a saltine cracker. You can make additional batches while the first batch is baking. The parchment paper can be re-used for additional batches.

Comments: "This recipe only takes about 5 minutes to mix and roll out - super easy!!"

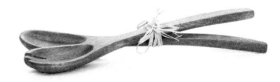

Wild Mushroom Cabbage Rolls

Ingredients:

- ¹/₂ cup pine nuts (pignolia) or favorite nuts
- 1 tablespoon olive oil
- 1 cup mushrooms – porcini, chanterelles, morels or button
- ¹/₄ cup chopped shallots
- 2 cloves garlic – minced
- 1 teaspoon sea salt
- 2 cups cooked brown rice
- 1 pound green cabbage leaf

Serving Size: 8

Toast pine nuts at 375 ° for 5 minutes.

Heat oil in a medium skillet and sauté mushrooms, shallots, garlic and salt until mushroom are limp. Stir in pine nuts and brown rice and let cool.

Wash individual cabbage leaves, steam for 1 minute and let cool.

Preheat oven to 375 °.

Stack 2-3 cabbage leaves one on top of the other and spoon 1/8 of the rice filling onto the stacked leaves. Roll the cabbage leaves around the filling and place in an oiled casserole dish, seam side down. Cover lightly with foil and bake at 375 ° for 20-30 minutes

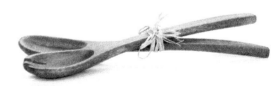

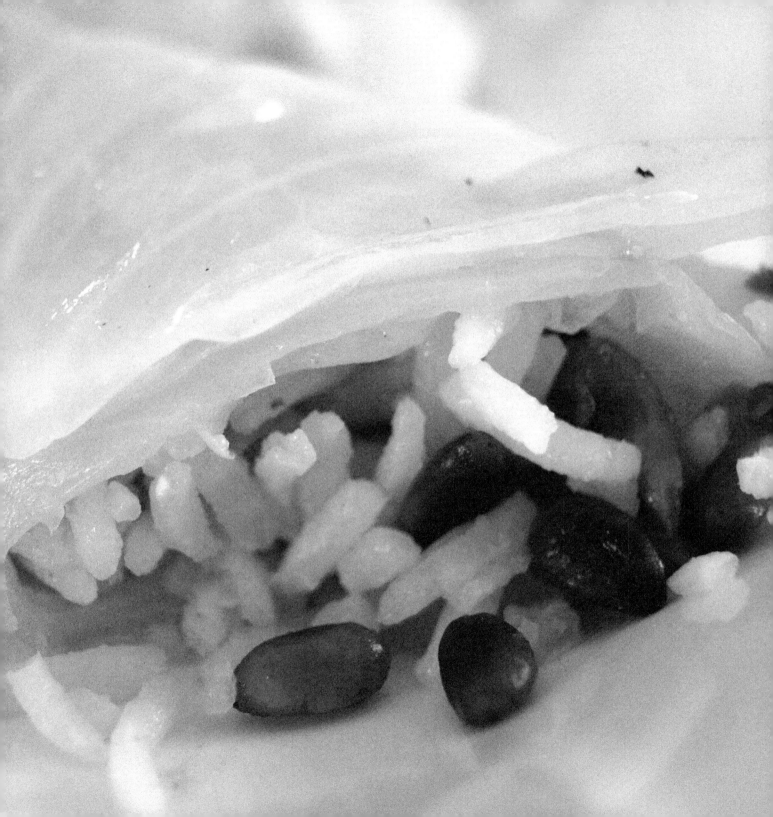

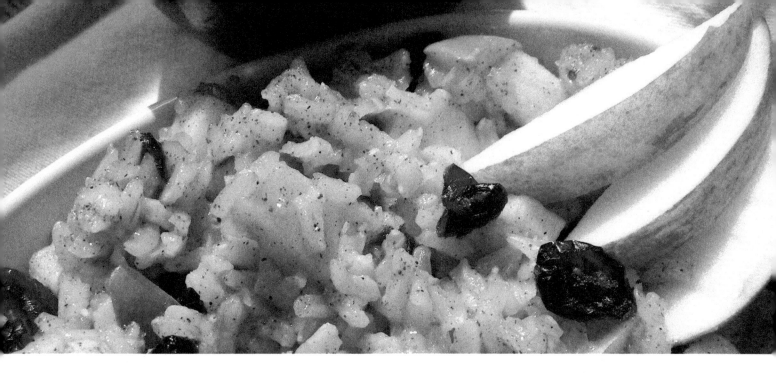

Yummy Brown Rice with Apple

Ingredients:

1   cup cooked brown rice

1   apple – diced

1   tablespoon raisins – or more if desired

1/4   teaspoon salt

1/2   teaspoon cinnamon

1   teaspoon coconut oil

2   teaspoon honey

Serving Size: 1

Mix all the ingredients together in a small casserole dish. Heat in oven 350° for 15 minutes till heated through. It is delicious.

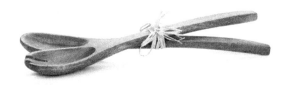

Encouragement for Fasting – 21 Daily Devotions

Written by Rhonda Sutton

Before You Start

For many years, I associated fasting with people in the Bible or extreme situations. When the subject of fasting appeared in this study, I had a profound thought: "This is too hard!" Then the Holy Spirit began to work in my heart and mind about fasting. He wouldn't let me alone. I had gone for years without ever sensing His desire for *me* to fast. As I read through the chapter on fasting, it seemed that everywhere I turned there were articles and books on fasting "jumping out" at me. Instead of dismissing these "coincidences", I decided to pray. Questions came to my mind. "Was the Lord asking *me* to fast? Couldn't I do something else for the Lord? Was this really necessary?" I knew that I did not have the will power to fast. He spoke very gently to my heart and said, "Keep your focus on *Me*. If you will walk with *Me* daily, *I will* give you the strength and grace for fasting". Then He said something that took me by surprise, "Claim this expression of love, obedience and faith, as a "done deal", *now*, even before you start the first day of fasting." Wow! This was too big. I was tempted to remind the Lord of my lack of self-discipline. He was asking me to trust *Him* during a fasting journey and submit to Him. I really did not want to refuse His loving invitation. He wanted me to focus on Him and His power, not on me and my weakness. I chose to fast to *please Him and to depend on Him alone each day*. I decided to go from fear of fasting to a deeper faith and freedom in Christ. The Lord faithfully has brought me through the "Daniel Fast" twice victoriously. Please prayerfully consider consecrating yourself by fasting. If you choose the "Daniel Fast", I will send a daily message to encourage you as you "fast by faith". We can do this together!

Day 1

Whether this is the first time fasting or the beginning of another fast, it all begins with the first day. We have chosen the Daniel Fast in a desire to draw closer to God through fasting. "This is the day the Lord has made, let us rejoice and be glad in it". We can be glad because He is going to help us with whatever comes our way today. We can be confident because nothing is too hard for the Lord Jesus!

You have prayed about fasting. It is important to ask for strength during the fast. The Holy Spirit is within us and we can depend on Him as our body begins to respond to the fasting process. When our stomachs growl today, we can rest and abide in the grace and truth that He is there helping us get through these challenges. Set aside some time during the usual meal time to pray and meditate on a favorite scripture passage. It is good to start a journal. Be sure to drink plenty of water so that the toxins and wastes can be easily flushed from your system.

Day 2

The stomach has a capacity that is just waiting to be filled. That's why you're experiencing such hunger. God has built into your body an automatic response. When your "tank is empty", you want to fill it. Because of that mechanism, we get in the habit of thinking often about food. Morning, mid-morning, noon, mid-afternoon, evening and even late evening, we go looking for things to satisfy our appetite. Yet during this fast, our focus is to be on a different capacity. We are to hunger for a deeper relationship with our loving Lord. After all, our fellowship with God is even more satisfying than food. So each time you sense that hunger, turn your mind to spiritual things. Recognize your need for God's love, mercy, wisdom and strength. Just think how wonderful it will be to concentrate, those five or six times a day, on God instead of food! That is the beauty of fasting.

Day 3

The marvels of fasting are starting to work on your body. Cells and tissues are releasing those toxins that have built up in your system. This is a very healthy change for you. But if you're not careful, you'll feel the effects of those toxins as they wind their way towards elimination. For example, you could have a really bad headache or even some muscle tension. Therefore, the best thing you can do is to drink plenty of water. That will help flush those toxins on out of your body. Even if you don't feel thirsty, drink some more.

While you're drinking lots of water and eliminating these poisons from your body, this is a good time to also seek for inner purity. Jesus said we are to thirst for righteousness (Matt. 5:6). During this fast, you may find improper personal attitudes and motivations coming to light. Let the Holy Spirit deal with those, just as if they were poison. You'll feel better!

Day 4

Did you know your body expects and depends on routine? As the day dawns, you desire nourishment. At mid-day, you seek more energy. At the close of the day, it's time to replenish your reserves. But on this day of fasting, let those signals turn your attention to a different kind of nourishment: the Word of God.

Truths from the Bible actually feed your soul. They make you stronger, wiser and spiritually healthy. So each time you think of food today, divert your thoughts to scripture. If you have your Bible nearby, read a significant section and ask God's Spirit to use it as divine nourishment. If you can't have a Bible with you during the day, then select a verse or two that you can memorize and carry with you. During your normal meal times, meditate on those verses and let them nurture your spiritual vitality. Use your hunger as a tool to help you grow stronger with the Lord.

Day 5

Today will probably be a difficult one physically. Your stomach will be aching for attention and your body will complain that it's not getting the treatment it craves. Yet this denial of self can be a very good thing. It throws into stark contrast the way your spirit has probably felt in the past. There were times when your spiritual life was not being fed and you paid attention primarily to your physical desires. On this day, however, the tables are turned. It's time for your Lord to be in the spotlight. He wants your focus to be more on Him and the quality of your relationship. It's alright if your flesh suffers a little today. It's worth the price if your walk with Jesus is prospering.

God hungers for you and desires a deep bond with you, one that goes beyond casual discipleship. He wants to be Number One in your life. As your body reminds you of its hunger, let that point you to God's passionate love for you.

Day 6

It is fatiguing to fight against the desires of the flesh, isn't it? Food is pleasurable to the senses and your body is crying out for some gratification. This is a good time to remind yourself that the purpose of this fast is to bring pleasure to the Lord, not your flesh. As you place your physical desires to the side and concentrate on your love relationship with God, the Lord is pleased. He has wanted to draw nearer to you and this is the opportunity for you both to be closer together.

According to James 4:8, when we draw near to God, He actually moves closer to us spiritually. Are you ready for that kind of encounter with the Creator? Perhaps you've already sensed a renewed intimacy with the Lord. If so, take some time today to praise the Lord. What a privilege it is to have a personal rapport with the Almighty!

Day 7

Your body is adapting to the lack of food. Your stomach is beginning to shrink and your cells are shedding those toxins. But today let's not think about what's happening with your body. Let's focus instead on your soul. A fast can become a time of heightened spiritual awareness. During this experience, let God speak to you about pollutants from this world that have imbedded themselves in your life. Are there attitudes, beliefs or viewpoints that negatively affect your relationship with God and with others?

Getting rid of worldly filth can be even more challenging than fasting. Today, ask the Lord to search your heart and help you in identifying those things that need to change. Confess those sins to the Savior and let him cleanse your heart. He will wash away the impurities, leaving you free once again to walk in the truth. This encounter with God may not be easy but you certainly don't want to avoid it. After this period of repentance, you'll feel so much better. When you take a bath or shower today, praise the Lord that He is cleansing you inside and rejoice as water washes away dead skin cells and eliminates odors. It is great to feel "clean" before the Lord! Praise His Name!

Day 8

For many of us, food has been a stronghold. It has exerted a power over us. We would schedule our days around eating, turn to snacks for comfort, and even hide from the pressures of the world inside our fortress of food. But no more! The walls of that stronghold are crumbling around us. We are now free! Doesn't it feel wonderful to know that food is not your master?

As you experience freedom, this is a prime opportunity to think about your friends and family who may be imprisoned by other strongholds. Food is not the only prison that we can build. Our loved ones may be dominated by drugs, alcohol, pornography, clothes, possessions, etc. What can you do about it? Turn your meal times today into moments of intercession. Take your mind off yourself and pray for those who are unknowingly in bondage. Ask the Lord to help them become free, just as He's helped you during this fast.

Day 9

During a fast, we become painfully aware of our weaknesses. Yes, we have hunger pangs and other aches that remind us of our mortal condition. But even more than that, we begin to see how weak we are inwardly. Our strength of will is challenged and we feel that we may fail in our resolve to fast. Our feelings are no longer dampened by the pleasures of food and we are shocked by some of our reactions to life. The only bright hope in all this is the Lord. When we are weak, He is strong.

God never expects you to achieve life's goals on your own. He designed you to need Him. That's why He's provided promises for you and me. He has an opened an account in your name and it's full of strength, wisdom, perseverance, joy, peace and love. All we have to do is access it through faith. This email is a gentle reminder to you that you're not alone in this journey. The Lord's promises are only a breath away.

Day 10

Friends and family may tell you that this fast doesn't make any sense. You may have even had such thoughts from time to time. But fasting is not a normal experience. It is a planned opportunity to "Trust in the LORD with all your heart, and lean not on your own understanding" (Prov. 3:5).

This far into the fast, you are probably being tempted to rationalize your way back to eating. You hear the voices of caring friends telling you to put an end to this practice. Or you "hear your body", telling you to cease fasting and get back to normal life. Actually, you find yourself at a crossroads. Will you listen to others or will you trust in the Lord and His strength? Will you yield to your body or to the encouraging whispers of the Holy Spirit? Let me cheer you on today: don't give up! Listen to the Lord, not to the world nor to the flesh. God will give you the support and perseverance that you need. You can do it!

Day 11

During these days of fasting, God has undoubtedly been teaching you things about yourself and about Himself. It's because of your physical discomforts that you've been made aware of your deepest desires and attitudes. Whereas those things remained hidden while your flesh was being satisfied, they've now been revealed and brought into the light. You've talked with the Lord and have attained a new depth of relationship. Isn't that exciting? Perhaps today you'll want to discuss even further those issues with Him.

While it's encouraging to receive fresh insights, they're not intended for you alone. It's good to share truth with those you love, with those who need to hear about God's love and faithfulness. You may know someone close to you who is discouraged and can't see the light of God. They're going through a dark time. Why not share with them what God has shown you. It could make a difference in their lives.

Day 12

As you continue down this pathway of fasting, you'll find that it's truly a sweet journey. You're experiencing victory and a new measure of health. It is important, however, to lay down some markers along the road. Someday you'll want to return to those markers and recall the successes you've had with God. There are a couple of ways to do this. The first is to choose some good Bible verses that you can associate with this time of fasting and triumph. Memorize them today and then meditate on them in the last half of your commitment.

You may also want to write a letter to God, expressing your appreciation for His strength and wisdom during this difficult time. You can mention to Him all that you've learned and the ways you've grown. Tuck that letter away in your Bible or in your bedside table. Later, you'll enjoy reflecting on all that God has done for you.

Day 13

Some days of fasting are harder than others. It's kind of like running a race. Sometimes you feel you've gotten your "second wind" while other times you feel near fatigue. How are you doing today? It's probably fairly difficult for you to keep going at this point. And that's precisely when you need to turn your gaze away from yourself and towards Jesus.

Take a look today at Hebrews 12:1-2. Jesus endured physical pains that we can hardly begin to imagine. He may have been tempted to give up, to stop his commitment to die on the cross. But Jesus didn't quit. He looked forward towards the end goal. He knew that joy and victory were just across the finish line. Won't you do the same today? Look ahead to the worthy accomplishment you'll have made. Contemplate the thrill of being victorious.

Then ask the Father to help you persevere, in the same way He helped Jesus remain on the cross. This can literally be a life-changing experience.

Day 14

As you complete this second week of fasting, take the time to complete an inventory. No, don't list everything you wish you could have eaten. It's time to jot down the values and priorities that you've seen hiding deep in your heart. What things have revealed themselves as being important to you? After noting your top ten treasures, turn your attention to the Lord. What would you say are His top ten priorities? Does your list align with His?

This is one of the greatest challenges to a child of God: submitting our cherished values to Him. As we do this, our number one passion in life will be to glorify God. Isn't that actually why you're committed to this fast? You want the Lord to be glorified through your body, mind and spirit. Therefore, ask the Holy Spirit today to fill you, to control you, so that all you do will be for the glory of God.

Day 15

Week Three! Praise the Lord! It's exciting that you have persevered, that God has helped you make it thus far. Whatever you do, don't stop drinking plenty of water. Keep yourself well hydrated. That's the key to staying healthy during this period of fasting.

Can you peer off into the distance, towards the end of this week? There is a finish line and it's already coming into view. Don't think of it as being far away. In fact, see yourself as actually completing the fast. View the moment, by faith, when you cross the goal and seal your victory. Consider it today to be a "done deal." There is no question that you will make it. Gaze on that coming success, knowing that you'll get there by walking in the Spirit, not in the flesh. As you enter this final chapter of your journey, ask the Lord to reveal Himself in a fresh way. Keep listening for his gentle whispers of encouragement.

Day 16

Would you say that these past two weeks have been a time of sacrifice? Absolutely! In fact, you have been a living sacrifice, just as Paul mentioned in Romans 12:1-2. Pause for a moment and read this passage anew. Remind yourself of what you have been experiencing. You have presented your body to the Lord in order to make it more pure and acceptable to Him. This has been a time of genuine worship. Also, you have undergone a transformation of your mind. You've discovered a fresh hunger for God and new desires for spiritual health.

As you move forward in this final week of fasting, let this be a time of celebration. You have much for which to be thankful. God has proven His faithfulness to you. And you are enjoying a new level of health, not just outwardly but inwardly. Let your praise show! May others see that you're walking in victory because of your mighty Lord.

Day 17

This fast has probably been unlike anything you've ever experienced. You've battled with your own flesh, wrestled with your feelings and altered your daily habits. Has anything taken you by surprise? Perhaps you didn't know how much this would affect your inner life. Or you've discovered a new strength that you didn't think you had. In any case, you've had some wonderful, unanticipated revelations. You've discovered a new depth of truth.

One of the reasons you've had these experiences is because you've been spending more time with Jesus, the Truth. Hasn't it been magnificent? Instead of eating in your "normal routine", you've been making healthy choices, talking to and listening to the Spirit. But what will you do once the fast is completed? Will you continue to have those precious moments with the Lord? Now is the time to start planning how you will carve out moments with God, once your life returns to its normal pace. This is a precious treasure that you don't want to lose.

Day 18

Why have you been fasting? That may seem to be a silly question, now that you're so close to reaching your goal. But it's important to determine your motivation. Was it solely because you wanted to lose weight? Or were you primarily driven by the desire to detoxify your body and experience increased health? I hope it's been more than that. The purest impulse for fasting can be found in 1 Corinthians 13:1-3. Love is the driving force that won't fall flat or take you down a dead end road. By fasting out of a deep love for God, you discover how crucial it is to have a solid relationship with the Lord.

Weight can fluctuate with time. It can't be your firm source of hope. And your health is not guaranteed. Things can change in a heartbeat. The only thing that you can count on is your Savior. Jesus said that he would never leave us or forsake us. In fact, he's with you today, ready to help you as you near the end of this fast. Praise the Lord! Please meditate and "chew on" on 1 Corinthians 13 today. Spend time "loving on" the Lord today and receive His wonderful love with deeper appreciation in a fresh way.

Day 19

You have had to tell yourself "no" so many times during the past couple of weeks. Your body has repeatedly asked for food and you've had to stay firm in your resolve. But this fast hasn't been about rules, right? Fasting is about freedom! It's about telling your body that it won't be your master. Yea! You aren't obligated to obey its impulses. You have only one Master and that is Jesus. With that kind of freedom, there is joy. Do you feel that deep sense of peace and fulfillment today? You have issued a declaration of independence from your fleshly desires. The skirmishes have been frequent, yet you've come through them victoriously. Look up Galatians 5:1 and read it out loud. Christ has made us free, free indeed! We are not slaves to our appetites any longer. Let us walk in this freedom and hold on to the truth with the strength of our beloved Master.

With that level of success, it's time to sing an anthem of freedom. You are stronger in your faith, purer in heart, and healthier in your body. Take the time today to actually celebrate and sing to the Lord. Make up a song that proclaims to God how much you appreciate your freedom in Christ. Sing your favorite praise songs in sweet worship to our King!

Day 20

Oh my! Tomorrow is the day! Are you getting really excited about completing the fast? It's going to be a day of glorious victory. So what are you going to do about it? Treat it like a normal day? I hope not. You need to have a special celebration, just like we do on Independence Day. You may not have any fireworks to shoot off, but you can do the next best thing. Prepare your spiritual sparklers!

Today is the time to plan your celebration event. Pick out all those favorite Bible verses that articulate what you want to say to God and to others. Have them lined out so you can give a litany of praise to the Lord. Do you have some preferred praise songs? Get the words together and have them ready to use. It's time for you to celebrate your independence, your freedom. You have not been a slave to food during this fast. Rejoice!

Day 21

You did it! Don't you feel like jumping up and down? This is truly an exciting moment. And yet I know what you're thinking. Even though you've been victorious, all you feel like doing is pointing to the Lord. He's the One who's given you the strength each day. All praise goes to Him.

As you celebrate today, think back to all the obstacles you had to overcome. God gave you everything you needed to do the impossible. He supplied wisdom, encouragement and power. If it's at all possible, go for a walk today with God. With each step, count your multitude of blessings. God has been incredibly good to you during this season of fasting. Now go tell someone what the Lord has meant to you during this time of testing. Proclaim His goodness. Please read Ephesians 3:16-21 and enjoy your victory lap!

You've made it! Congratulations! The Lord is exalted and He is your eternal reward!

Daniel Fast Commitment

I commit to following the Daniel Fast for the following dates:

_____ to _____

The purpose of this fast is to draw closer to God through prayer and Bible study, and to abstain from certain foods for discipline.

I also commit to pray for those who are joining me on this physical and spiritual journey.

Name _____

Date _____

Accountability Partner (optional) _____

Daniel Fast Commitment

I commit to following the Daniel Fast for the following dates:

_____ to _____

The purpose of this fast is to draw closer to God through prayer and Bible study, and to abstain from certain foods for discipline.

I also commit to pray for those who are joining me on this physical and spiritual journey.

Name _____

Date _____

Accountability Partner (optional) _____

OTHER BOOKS AND MATERIALS
BY ANNETTE AND DR. RICHARD COUEY:

Available on the Designed Healthy Living website.

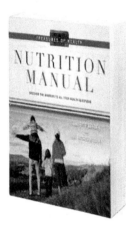

Nutrition Manual

Are you tired of reading book after book to find the answers to your health concerns? Look no further! At your fingertips is a complete resource for information on nutrition and a healthy lifestyle. Treasures of Health Nutrition Manual combines information on the nourishment from God-created foods with truths about the value of vitamins to help you create a healthy, happy home and body. This book, along with the other two books will elaborate on the treasure trove of information in Scripture about wellness and nutrition. It will also direct you to the knowledge and understanding of:

- How God designed your body.
- What foods are going to deliver nutrition.
- The value of vitamins.
- The ultimate treasures of being happy and healthy

Treasures of Healthy Living

Everyone loves a treasure hunt. The hunt can be almost as rewarding as the final treasure! Follow the clues on our map and discover the answers to a healthy life full of vitality. This study will unveil the counterfeits and substitutions currently robbing us of energy and zest for living. Then it will fill the void with overflowing riches of health. This Bible Study will give you and your group the tools needed to reclaim health in the balance God designed. This study speaks to a new generation hungry for answers and looking for God's design.

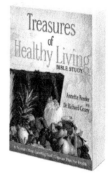

Available soft cover and Kindle

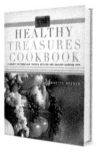

Healthy Treasures Cookbook

This bounty of recipes and cooking tips will encourage you to bring healthy treasures back to the dinner table. Surprise and delight will abound as you please your family with these tasty meals that will also contribute to their health and well-being. Whether you are a beginner or novice in the kitchen, this book covers it all.

Available soft cover